WHEN TREES WERE GREEN

'How about getting out of doors for a while, Robin?' It was a balmy afternoon. Robin was looking out on the gardens as Dr Monaghan passed room No. 12.

Robin was wrapped in blankets with an anorak tucked over his dressing gown. Tremulously, I navigated the wheelchair into the lift, through the swing doors of the Reception area and out into the sunshine.

Robin was ecstatic.

For over an hour, he explored a forgotten world of sunlight, movement and colour. His responses were intense. The delight in the feel of a whispering breeze on his face. The warmth of sunshine on his skin.

When Trees Were Green

Inez Heron

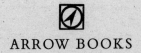

ARROW BOOKS

Arrow Books Limited
3 Fitzroy Square, London WP 6JD

An imprint of the Hutchinson Publishing Group

London Melbourne Sydney Auckland
Wellington Johannesburg and agencies
throughout the world

First published in Great Britain by Michael Joseph 1978
Arrow edition 1979
© 1978 by Inez Heron

Made and printed in Great Britain
by The Anchor Press Ltd
Tiptree, Essex

ISBN 0 09 919610 7

For my son, who survived.
In memory of R. W. Shaw, who died;
and to W. L. who *Touched*
                    The fractured shell
                    With tenderness
                    —and gently
                    Held it
                    Till it turned
                    To Gold

Contents

Acknowledgements

Grateful acknowledgement is made to the following for permission to reprint previously published material:

Alfred A. Knopf for words from *Sand and Foam*, by Kahlil Gibran; copyright 1926 by Kahlil Gibran; renewal copyright 1954 by Administrators C.T.A. of Kahlil Gibran Estate and Mary G. Gibran (page 26); Katherine Kavanagh for words from Patrick Kavanagh's *To a Child*, published by Martin Brian & O'Keeffe Ltd. (page 35); Basil Payne for words from *An Answer to Allegory* (page 38); Release Records for words from Peadar Kehoe's *Slaney Valley* (page 39); Denis Johnston for words from *The Old Lady Says 'No'* (page 61); Tro Essex Music for words from *The Bells of Hell* (page 83); Faber & Faber Ltd for words from W. H. Auden's *Musée des Beaux Arts* (page 141); Macmillan and Co Ltd for words from W. B. Yeats' *Easter 1916* (page 209); and the *Sunday Times* for words from Harold Hobson (page 219)

PROLOGUE

'He could not die when trees were green,
For he loved the time too well.'
John Clare (*The Dying Child*)

We were a pretty ordinary family really. Six of us, living an uneventful suburban life.

There was Bob, my husband. He was a bank manager; reserved and dependable with high integrity and exceptional tolerance. A gentle 'family' man. Our ten-year marriage balanced well, for I thrived on activity and involvement with people. Free-lance journalism, combined with some radio scriptwriting and broadcasting, gave me the outlet of expression which I needed. And, I felt, my family benefited as a result.

When Trees Were Green is a story that began eight years ago. It recounts the illness of our eldest son, Robin. During the long months of vigil at his bedside, I kept notes day by day; notes of my thoughts, of the little events which occurred, of Robin's vacillating condition. Subconsciously perhaps I was harvesting a diary of memories for the time when, after Robin's death, those jottings would be all that remained of him.

Some impulse drove me to edit those scribblings into a book. At the start, I was resurrecting phantoms of the past in an attempt to exorcise them. Then the importance of Toxocariasis began to dominate.

Robin's illness had originally been diagnosed as a lymphosarcoma, a cancer of the lymph glands. It was an understandable error of identification for Toxocariasis was, at that time, considered to be comparatively rare in humans.

However, one of the British medical journals published a paper, in September 1970, on the subject of Toxocaral infection. It concluded by stating that although Toxocariasis was scarcely known as a human infection until 1960, it is widespread and sometimes a cause of death. The public health problems of the infection are grave and and need prompt attention.

Compiling these notes was not easy writing. The effort and time expended were demanding. The emotional pressure was traumatic but a compulsion drove me on to the end.

ONE

June, July

'...for the world, which seems
To lie before us like a land of dreams,
So various, so beautiful, so new,
Hath really neither joy, nor love, nor light,
Nor certitude, nor peace, nor help for pain;
And we are here as on a darkling plain...'
Matthew Arnold (*Dover Beach*)

Robin was eight years old when it all began.

Billie, aged seven, came next in line. Then there was Helen, our daughter. She was five and mentally retarded. Michael was the baby. Eleven weeks after his birth, our lives changed irrevocably.

It was a Sunday morning, in June 1970.

The trouble had started about a fortnight before with Robin having occasional abdominal pains, with isolated days of feeling in poor form. The pains became more frequent. Finally, that Sunday morning, when the pain was very severe, we called our GP. There were none of the classical symptoms of appendicitis, the GP said. No vomiting or nausea. No abnormal temperature.

'I think it's appendix trouble,' he commented. 'Anyway, I'd like a surgeon to see him right away.'

The GP made a telephone call to Holy Innocents' Hospital.

'Oriel Verkonnen is on call today. He's an excellent man,' he remarked, covering the mouthpiece while waiting for Robin's booking to be confirmed. 'I was at University with him. A very good chap.'

I filled up the routine form at Admissions.

Name: Robin Heron
Age: 8 years 8 months
Religion: Roman Catholic
Parents: Bob and Inez Heron

I signed another document, authorising the administration of a general anaesthetic.

Then a nurse led us through a maze of corridors and up in a lift to St Canice's Ward on the first floor. It was suffused in sunlight. Glass-partitioned cubicles opened off a main passage.

Ward Sister came out from her centrally-located Station which gave a panoramic view of her whole domain. She was a striking dark-eyed girl in blue, her black hair conventionally knotted up under her lace cap. Her badge identified her as 'Sr White'.

She showed Robin to his room. A tiny wisp of a child watched us from the other bed.

'Appendicitis is the commonest cause of emergency surgery. You'll be home again in less than a fortnight,' I said to Robin. I had no premonition of fear as he lay on the hospital bed, wide-eyed with interest.

'Well, I suppose they've plenty of practice, then,' he replied philosophically.

'They've been removing appendices for nearly a hundred years, I gather,' I continued reassuringly. Before we'd left home, I had hurriedly glanced at our medical dictionary. I liked to check facts; possibly a legacy from journalistic researching. I also had developed the habit of talking to the boys as young adults. The results might have been regarded as a certain degree of precocity; I preferred to think of it as early mental maturing.

A doctor breezed in, an intern with a shaggy mane of hair and thick-soled desert boots. He examined Robin, asked a few questions, then made abstruse markings on a chart. The ball-pointed nib traced strange symbols on the printed outline of a human body. He gathered up his papers and removed them.

Gone were the griping pains which had recurred and troubled Robin since his return from our family holidays, several days before. Now he only vaguely experienced a sensation of soreness when pressure was applied to the right side of his abdomen.

Over an hour later, I left. It was after mid-day and Robin was contentedly chatting with some boys who had wandered in to the two-bedded cubicle.

'There isn't much point in waiting,' Sr White said. 'It will be a little while before we have him ready for surgery and he'll be muzzy when he comes back from Theatre. If you telephone about four o'clock, we should have news for you.'

Holy Innocents' was a half-hour drive from home and Bob and I motored back there in the late afternoon.

The space where Robin's bed had been was empty.

'He isn't back yet,' Robin's tiny room-mate volunteered in a childish treble. We left a Get-Well card on the locker along with a few favourite books.

Sr White assured us she would be in contact later.

Evening came. We still had heard nothing.

It was night-time when the GP phoned. His voice disturbed me. Not just his tiredness which percolated down the line, but a hesitancy, a concern.

'Sorry not to have been in touch earlier. But Robin was rather longer in Theatre than was expected.' I let him continue, uninterrupted. 'It's a little more serious than an appendix, I'm afraid, Mrs Heron.'

Confusion flooded over me. What was he trying to say? What serious condition could surgery reveal in an eight-year-old child? Children didn't have gall-stones or ulcers or slipped spinal discs? . . . or did they?

His voice drifted on. Words; alien, unfamiliar yet ominous.

'Tumours . . . growths . . . of course, probably benign . . . tests will tell . . .'

I interrupted him. 'Cancer? You don't mean cancer?'

I awaited his denial but it didn't come. He spoke of hope, of children having a good chance.

I broke in. 'But, doctor, what sort of cancer? Where? I mean, Robin's been in such good health . . .' Maybe I had misunderstood him.

'There are different sorts of cancers. Many different types. Mr Verkonnen will explain it all to you. I'll phone you on Wednesday. We'll have the results of the tests by then.'

Wednesday. Three days to Judgement Day. Apocalyptical Three Days in the Tomb. Then Resurrection?

No! Already somewhere in the rambling complex of hospital buildings, neat little containers of Robin's body tissue would have been labelled, awaiting the technicians' attention. Tomorrow someone would start another Monday morning's work. Someone would potter over plates and slides. Dissect; analyse; process. And then, three days later, a pathologist would note his findings on the appropriate form. Give his verdict and sign it.

Robin's sentence would be passed. Had already been passed; for, malignant or benign, reason told me that nothing could now change the reality. Nothing.

The nightmare had begun.

My hands shook convulsively as I replaced the receiver. Instinct banished conditioned inhibitions. My head dropped on to my knees. My arms locked around my body. I rocked and moaned in a grief as raw and naked as aboriginal woman of Earth's last primeval tribe.

Then the dry sobbing gave way to panic. I dashed from the telephone to where Bob sat watching television.

'Well?' he looked up expectantly. 'What's happened?'

And incoherently, my hands covering my face, I tried to babble out the awful message.

What had I expected? That overnight Robin would have wasted? Yellowed? That Father Time, armed with scythe, would be peering out from behind the Disneyland cubicle curtains? Death playing with Bambi and Dumbo in their happy-ever-after world of fantasia?

Rhetorical questions surfaced from the dark corners of my mind. Of course, Robin looked the same. He was awake and restless, irritable from the discomfort of the IV drip which carried fluid into a vein in his left hand.

I read the notations on his chart. '*4.00 a.m. crying; morphine. Temperature: normal*'.

That normality almost assuaged my fears.

The day after surgery, the abdominal bandages were replaced by a small dressing. The next day, the IV tube was removed and the parched dryness of forty-eight hours' thirst was relieved by sips of water.

'It's great! Two teaspoonfuls of water. I can leave it in my mouth and swoosh it round and enjoy it.' Robin spat out with relish into a dish.

A cage, draped in a sheet, covered his lower trunk and legs. A plaster pad on his hand almost concealed the bruising where the anaesthetic had been administered. Everything seemed so ordinary that a trickle of hope filtered back into my life.

Tomorrow we would know the verdict.

But we didn't hear.

All day we waited. At Holy Innocents' no one volunteered any information. The GP didn't telephone.

En route back from the hospital that Wednesday night, we called at his home. His wife answered the bell, hair wound up in rollers, naked feet white in floppy mules.

I apologised for calling so late. She was understanding. In the shaft of light from the open hall-door we stood; two figures in a spotlight.

She fumbled for words. 'No. The doctor didn't hear from Mr Verkonnen today, Mrs Heron. I'm certain of that.'

Dejection fell over me like a cloak. She seemed to sense it. Hesitantly, as though fearing intrusion, she went on.

'We're all praying for you. For your little boy—that he'll be all right. The children are remembering him in the Family Rosary each night.'

I murmured my thanks.

Prayer. It was all that was left now to insulate us against the future.

We had made our initial mistake when we first mentioned Robin's suspected condition outside the family circle. The telephone rang ceaselessly. Enquiries. Promises of Rosaries, of triduums, Masses and novenas.

I clung to the kindness of friends. To the hope that a belief in God afforded me. I clung to the atavistic faith in Omnipotence which had supported Irish Catholicism through centuries of religious repression.

'With God all things are possible.'

'Faith can move mountains.'

'More things are wrought by prayer than this world dreams of.'

Each passing night, I drew on the strength of assurance of God's love, unconcerned by the source of origin of such quotations. The Old Testament? The Gospels? The Koran? Prophetic dreams or poetic visions? It didn't matter. They comforted me a little.

By day, I developed a talent for acting and played out a charade of calm optimism.

Mornings. Sunny mornings.

I parked the car on the wide concrete apron and exchanged greetings with the Hall Porter. He didn't check my visiting card, for already my appearance was familiar to him. This new routine was becoming our way of life.

Visiting hours were almost unrestricted: two visitors at a time with a patient, from mid-morning until eight o'clock. We divided the day into three zones. I spent a couple of hours with Robin each morning. In the afternoon, my mother called to see him. A labour dispute had left Bob unemployed along with thousands of others and he was trying, unsuccessfully, to get a job. After tea, he joined me for an evening session of jigsaw-making, and card playing, with a cluster of children from St Canice's Ward. About an hour after the day staff went off duty, we left Robin to settle for the night.

He had had four blood tests since his operation. No one told us why or gave us the results. No one told us anything. But my faith in God and in the medical staff was absolute. They were doing what was best.

Robin's progress was marked by complaints. His voice grew strident with irritation. 'I hate the bed pan. Sometimes the wet gets on the bed and they cover the damp part with nappies. It's horrible!' he protested.

The cursory wash which was administered no longer satisfied his fastidiousness. 'Once you're getting better, no one washes you. Could you bring in a bowl and mug so that I can clean my teeth and wash myself?' he asked.

We did. Half-sitting up in bed, he sloshed his way through his ablutions to his personal satisfaction, keeping up a running commentary on hospital events.

'I hate letting anyone near me now, because often it's with a needle for an injection. And it's awful.' He changed the subject abruptly. 'I've started to read again. Could you bring me in some more of my books, please? They help me to forget all this,' and he waved his toothbrush like a wand embracing the whole ward.

One morning, the priest brought the Eucharist to St Canice's patients. Later, Robin reported on his visit.

'The Holy Communion came in two chalices on a tray. A nun came first with a little red light and ringing a bell. Then the priest. He looked very young', he said.

'Newly ordained priests are often assigned to convents or schools or hospitals, as a first appointment,' I explained.

Robin went on. 'Did you see the Indian doctor, Mum? He wears his hair done up in a scarf. A sort of turban.'

'Maybe he's a Sikh. Their religion doesn't allow them to cut their hair, you see.'

He thought a moment. 'Funny thing, religion – isn't it?'

Activity on the passage. Nurses fluttered to the Staff Rest Room, to straighten caps, remove rings and other banned jewellery.

An outsize trolley, laden with files, was pushed from the Station to the swing-doors of St Canice's. A prelude to Ward Rounds. Presently, the team swung in. A phalanx of house surgeons and interns was preceded by the Consultant. I heard the name 'Mr Verkonnen'. Proffered files; stop-over at a selected bed; a few words to Sr White, and they moved on.

I hadn't seen Oriel Verkonnen before. He was fortyish – a physically beautiful tall man, with white-blond hair and satin gold skin.

Perfunctory introductions. Softly cadenced voice, remote and professional.

I looked at the hands that lightly touched Robin's abdomen; at the fingers which, gloved and sterile, had incised and probed on a routine appendectomic mission. Then paused; probed further. And discovered – what?

I didn't know.

Mr Verkonnen moved away in silence. A flurry of nurses bustled behind him, striving to catch his comments. Sr White made notes on the relevant files.

His slender figure had an aura of quiet authority. He continued down the ward, cosseted from the intrusive questions of relatives by his coterie of students.

Rounds finished, he paused at Robin's door. The entourage melted away. He beckoned to me. 'Could I have a word with you?'

We crossed the passage to a small ante-room located between the linen press and the sluice room. It was a sparsely furnished office; two chairs, a table and a telephone.

Someone spoke to him from the corridor. He turned back, his hand on the open door. Through the window, I glanced down at the car park. Coloured cellulose and polished chromium sparkled in the sunshine.

The door closed gently. Mr Verkonnen stood facing me. He didn't sit down and neither did I.

Haltingly, I queried, 'Did you have any results from Pathology?'
He nodded.

With nerves taut as coiled steel wire, I heard his reply. He added a few brief words.

I felt a dry burning behind my eyes; a tightening brace of pain clamped around my temples.

Robin had cancer.

As Robin began to recover from surgery, his spirits revived.

I wilted. Physically, I felt permanently tired. The hours of inactivity, of chatting and playing and entertaining him made me disproportionately weary. I was exhausted by day; restless at night.

Robin began to eat. 'I'd a super breakfast. Sausages and tea. The cornflakes aren't nice, though. They're put out in little bowls the night before, the other lads told me. That's why they're always soggy.'

More blood tests.

Robin could walk around the bed now, shakily on weak legs. His red hair clung greasily to his scalp. It had been rubbed with olive oil; a routine hospital procedure – hygienically necessary apparently but aesthetically unattractive.

He developed an aversion to the toilets. As with all the other wards, St Canice's had its own lavatories off the main corridor. There were four cubicles. The walls were garnished with brown smears of excreta from uncoordinated little fingers attempting to rid themselves of the residue of faulty wiping. Inaccurate marksmen contributed their share of splashes and puddles on the terrazzo floor. Although the lavatories were regularly scoured out, it was difficult to combat the choking of the bowls with paper. A confetti scattering of flittered tissue sprinkled the whole area.

'You'd want Wellington boots for going in there,' Robin commented. 'In fact, you could go fishing if you'd a rod and line – there are so many foreign bodies floating around.'

I smiled at his description and assured him that soon he would be home and back to normality.

The second week neared its end. Visitors came with presents, and Robin's moods vacillated from delight to dejection.

On Friday, Oriel Verkonnen made his customary Ward Round. He called me into the ante-room. I felt we had played the scene before. But I was wrong: this was new. He didn't waste words.

'I'll have to operate again.'

I choked. 'Why?'

'For Robin's sake. It would be beneficial to do a thorough exploration of the intestines.' His decision was authoritive.

I accepted his judgement. It represented hope and I clung to hope. It was all I had.

'When do you plan to do it?' I tried to steady my voice.

'On Monday next.'

Blood tests again. Medicines.

Waiting.

Because we were such regular visitors, the other boys at St Canice's accepted us and gravitated towards us. Robin became uneasy. He grew possessive of his books, his games and our company. He developed an antipathy towards some of the children, towards Danny and Rex and Cathal. Towards Tim and Aidan whom he heard but never saw.

. . . Everyone at Holy Innocents' knew Danny; ubiquitous, dark-eyed Danny. He was a paraplegic, noiselessly rolling through the maze of hospital passages in his wheelchair. His arms and hands were powerful; a strength developed through the necessity of propelling himself around.

He was twelve years old, with thick curly hair and sensitively chiselled features. From below the waist, his body was twisted and deformed. His legs, revealed sometimes when his rug slipped off, dangled limply – their growth stunted in size to those of a toddler.

Danny was refreshingly devoid of inhibitions. He navigated bed-ends and drip-stands with panache. His urine drained into a polythene bag which balanced on the empty footplate of his wheelchair. Occasionally, it fell to the ground, and he would smile disarmingly. 'Careful! Don't step on it, it will squelch!'

In the evenings, he joined us playing cards on Robin's bed. He had no sense of form. The most elementary games defeated him. He couldn't cope with the simplest jigsaws.

Once I gave him an adventure story. He opened the book enthusiastically, then looked away. His dark eyes were clouded as he handed it back to me. 'I can't read,' he explained simply.

Twelve-year-old Danny. Beautiful, intelligent, paraplegic. Stultified in development by his environment. He lived in a convent orphanage, a nurse told me, and he spent his holidays at Holy Innocents'. There was a hospital school but his attendance appeared to be irregular. Maybe his life expectancy was short and the authorities considered it kinder not to pressurise him needlessly. Yet it seemed tragic that the escapism of reading was denied him.

Sometimes Danny disappeared for a couple of days. He kept his few possessions in a carrier bag and moved into whatever vacant bed was available in whichever ward took his fancy. St Canice's was a favourite with him. Being surgical, there was a steady turnover of new arrivals. New faces and passing friendships. Diagnosis, surgery, recuperation, discharge. Danny alone remained. A semi-permanent resident.

Often Danny touched my body physically. Tactility was essential to his warm nature. He would roll up to Robin's bed in the evenings, expertly remove the arm-rest of his wheelchair and lean over until his head rested against my shoulder. His hands would hold my fingers, feel my hair, touch my cheek. Softly he would whisper, 'You're my Mummy. I'm going to call you Mummy. You're *my* Mummy and Daddy because you come to see me so often.' Robin would glare silently, barely concealing his resentment.

As Danny was lifted into bed at night, he would cling to the nurse and plead with her. 'Kiss me goodnight. Please, Nurse, please.' Reactions varied with the individual personalities. Some shied away uneasily, embarrassed at a possible manifestation of puberty. Others gave him a little sign of the loving for which he craved. Love does not exist until it is given away. Danny yearned to give.

One night, as he was lying in his cubicle, I passed by. A plaintive voice called me. 'Can I kiss you goodnight, Mummy, please?' My mouth touched his forehead. His lips brushed my cheek. "It is indeed misery if I stretch an empty hand and receive nothing; but it is hopelessness if I stretch a full hand and find none to receive."

Danny. Abandoned legacy of a forgotten love affair? It seemed so. Perhaps it was so . . .

. . . The day Rex arrived, a special bed had to be installed. Holy

26

Innocents' catered for children up to fifteen years old. Rex presumably qualified in age, but he was a wiry, lean six-footer and a generous length of leg protruded from the bottom of the small bed allocated to him. A battalion of blue-clad porters erected a full-size bed in a single cubicle near the Ward Station. These rooms were usually reserved for patients needing special care following surgery. Rex, correctly, was assessed as being an 'exceptional' case.

Immediately he'd settled in, he took over St Canice's Ward.

'Any dolly birds around?' he enquired hopefully, and soon was on flirtatious terms with the young probationer nurses.

He quickly organised a card school. He initiated the older boys into poker and arranged frequent forays at night to the ward kitchen where he brewed endless cups of instant coffee. Most of the information about other patients came via Rex. He was a bright talkative extrovert.

The day after his tonsillectomy, he held court to a host of leather-jacketed friends. In desperation, Sr White phoned for a porter to come; and Rex's visitors were reduced to the regulation twosome.

Each evening his parents called. His father, a small balding man, surreptitiously smoked illicit cigarettes and puffed the evidence out through the cubicle window. His mother was blonde and blousy; her voluptuous figure was magnificently corseted into controlled curvaceousness. Her vivacity was equalled by her loud enthusiastic laughter as, through the glass partition, she vetted the House Surgeons with frank appraising interest.

Rex made the prompt recovery one would have expected of him. With his departure, St Canice's lost some of its light . . .

. . . Cathal was the little waif who shared Robin's room. At some stage of each day he had visitors. If they didn't come in the afternoon, he would hover around the top of the stairs, peering down, waving vicariously at everyone who passed until some of the nurses shooed him back into St Canice's Ward. But his visitors never failed him. Occasionally, two hefty teenage girls with silky-seaweed hair and trendy colourful clothes arrived. More often, it was an elderly lady armed with a shopping bag of edibles and toys.

Cathal was a diminutive mouse of a boy with shaggy hair and ill-fitting trousers which hung loosely on his tiny frame. He usually wore a scarlet jumper. It accentuated his pallor.

27

As he sat on my knee, engrossed in playing with Robin and Bob, the sharp bones of his buttocks caused me to fidget. He wriggled round, looking up into my face, a slight squint in his pale-grey eyes.

'Me grannie'll be here soon,' he said. It wasn't a question but a self-reassuring statement. He talked about his parents, his brothers and sisters in their home in the city.

'We do live in the Corporation flats. We've the front room and two back rooms on the second floor. But me Daddy an' me Mammy can't come in for to see me like. They do be at home minding the babbies.'

'Mmm. It must be difficult for them,' I agreed gravely.

The truth was different. Cathal had no home. He lived in an orphanage in the country. His visitors were a city family who took him out to spend Christmas and summer holidays with them. Cathal had adopted them as his own.

Fantasy can effectively supplant reality when the reality is too hard to bear . . .

. . . The last cubicle on the passage was occupied by Tim. Though I rarely saw him, I frequently heard him at irregular intervals of day or evening; strange whooping cries which echoed along the corridor.

Tim was three years old, immobile in his cot. Only the faint movement of his head indicated that some acoustical vibration penetrated and registered in his brain. He was fed with a tube from a baby bottle. Through constantly lying on his side to avoid choking on his vomit, the shape of his face was no longer round, but sharply pointed. Occasionally, the heavy-lidded eyes fluttered half open, unfocused.

The nurses handled him with infinite tenderness. His luxuriant growth of baby-fine hair was brushed and combed. It lay, a dark nimbus, on the white sheet.

The cubicle was opposite the ward kitchen. Once, as I was coming out, I noticed a translucent tear that had slipped like a crystal from his unseeing eyes and dried on the pale skin of his cheek.

Can the living dead weep for forfeited life . . .?

. . . From physical appearances, it was difficult to assess Aidan's age. He was probably about seven, judging by the gaps where his milk teeth had fallen out. He was receiving treatment for hydrocephalus. His head was grossly enlarged. The eyes protruded from the tiny features of his face, lost under the great dome of the cranium. Pre-surgical preparation had left his scalp shorn of hair.

Aidan slept alone in a single cubicle. For endless hours during the day he would lie, partially propped up by pillows, seemingly unresponsive to his surroundings. The only view through the glass door in front of him, was the red sentinel of a fire extinguisher fixed to the wall. Sometimes he was lifted into a chair and placed on the balcony outside in the sunshine.

One afternoon, as he was sitting on the verandah near Robin's room, I heard intermittent snuffling. A strange sniffing sound, like a puppy trying to sneeze. Aidan's shoulders were shaking spasmodically. His head moved slightly. Apprehensive of interfering, I opened the French door. He couldn't turn, but he heard the noise. He stretched out his hand. I took it silently in mine and sat down on the concrete beside him, my legs tucked under me.

His cheeks were wet. His eyes blurred with tears. Gently I dried them with a tissue. A tremulous smile lit the distorted features. I spoke softly, still holding his hand in mine. Spoke of the children playing on the grass below; of the gulls wheeling high overhead, soaring effortlessly in a thermal current.

How much registered through the fluidic pressure on his brain, I couldn't tell, but gradually the snuffling crying ceased. Presently a nurse came and carried him back to his cubicle.

A woman had been watching from further down the balcony. She captured me before I could return to Robin, anxiety to participate written on her face. 'That poor child. Isn't he awful? When first I seen him, it gemme that big a shock that I had to sit down. I just had to sit down. I couldn't look at him.'

I turned away from her.

The night before Aidan's departure, his parents came to see him. His father, a red-faced cheerful man, organised a sing-song of traditional Irish favourites. A trickle of children, armed with towels en route from the washroom, drifted in. Aidan's face was alight with happiness.

Next morning, his mother collected his hold-all. She followed the nurse down the corridor, plodding heavily behind Aidan's wheel-chair. A shabby, weary woman, prematurely aged. An eight-hour journey lay ahead of her; a journey by rail and road to the north of

Co. Donegal. A journey in which there could be no escape from those eyes that would stare curiously, then look away in horror . . .

. . . Robin didn't know of Malcolm's existence. I never met him, but his mother taught me a salutary lesson in realism.

'*You just go on,*' she said, '*because you've no alternative.*'

I only met her once but the memory of her will remain with me forever. It was the morning after the Irish Mist Ball, a charitable social event. She was sitting in the hospital coffee bar drowning a mammoth hangover. By unwritten code of protocol, the secretarial and administrative staffs sat apart from the paramedics. The patients' visitors found what accommodation they could.

Robin was asleep and I had escaped for a few minutes to recharge my batteries in anticipation of the day ahead.

The dour coffee bar attendant clattered down the metal curtain of her counter, with no verbal warning of closing time.

'Christ!' said the red-headed woman at the next table. 'I needed another cup – and how!' It was her opening gambit for conversation.

The Irish Mist Ball was organised to raise funds for children suffering from cystic fibrosis. 'C.F.' children, she called them. She had given birth to two. One, a boy, had died a couple of years previously when aged ten. The other was Malcolm. Only her chain-smoking and the colourful expletives punctuating her conversation revealed the strain under which she lived.

'Malcolm is six now. He was admitted a few weeks ago for treatment. Just an infection. C.F. children are very susceptible to infection. However, he's responding to antibiotics.'

At home, he slept in a mist tent. 'It keeps the mucous in his lungs moist and he can cough it up and relieve his breathing. At the moment, he's having physiotherapy as well. That's why I'm here so early this morning. Jesus! I feel bloody awful!' She lit a cigarette. 'You see, Malcolm sets up a screaming when he sees the therapist on the passage. It's bang-bang-bang around his back and chest and he hates it.'

She drew heavily until the tip glowed red.

'My older boy took five months' hospitalisation to die. And the pain of therapy on his emaciated body was quite terrible. He'd cough and cough and up would come this mucous – thick as chewing gum.'

She inhaled again. 'With Malcolm, we knew his condition from the start. It's genetic, you know. They're born with it and they die from it. There's excessive mucous secretion. In Malcolm, it's in the lungs and intestines. The gut,' she explained.

'He takes a medicine with supplementary enzymes which help digestion. But his stools are very loose, something like diarrhoea most of the time. He's getting to the age when he's sensitive about it. So when he goes to the toilet, he takes his own aerosol spray to freshen the place. But there's always a terrible smell, both from the faeces and his breath. It's the medicine, I suppose.'

They had taken the eldest boy to Lourdes. 'Not that there's any cure as yet, for cystic fibrosis. There won't be until there's a breakthrough in genetic engineering. But Lourdes is a last-ditch stand for many of the parents. There's always the hope of a miracle. They feel that everything possible which could be done, has been done.'

She told me how her son had been terrified by the procedure at the Baths there. 'There's a special unit for children. A Piscine. It's a big tank of water channelled from St Bernadette's spring and manned by a team of voluntary helpers. They're very kind. But the children can't understand what it's all about. The strangers, the undressing, the chilly water. They're forcibly immersed in it up to the neck three times, and prayers are said in French for them. I just couldn't stand the screaming and the struggling. Couldn't bear it. That's why we're not taking Malcolm. I just haven't the faith or the courage any more.'

She stubbed out the dying cigarette and stood up. 'Christ! My bloody head!' She braced herself.

Involuntarily, I exclaimed, 'My God! You've got courage.'

She leaned towards me. Her voice suddenly seemed excessively weary. 'You're wrong. It's not courage, you know. It's endurance. You just go on because you've no alternative.'

Sunday evening came with an influx of visitors. Excited children revelled in popcorn, lemonade and crisps, and were reluctant to settle that night.

Sr White clipped a notice to Robin's bedrail. '*Keep fasting*'. He viewed it suspiciously.

I lied to reassure him. 'Possibly it means that they want to do tests. Food might interfere with the results.'

He accepted the explanation. 'You're probably right,' he agreed. 'I've seen them on other beds. They've three notices, actually. "*Keep fasting*". "*Clear fluids only*". "*Mixed fluids*". It's probably just for a check-up before I go home.'

I nodded.

Later, Sr White allayed my unease. 'He'll be going to Theatre under the impression it's for an X-ray. We'll give him an injection and he'll be drowsy before he leaves the ward. Don't worry about him.'

By the lift-shaft, the surgical roster for the following morning was pinned to a noticeboard, white typewritten paper on green baize. I had sometimes glanced at it as I passed.

That night I didn't stop to look at the list.

The operation was over when I called at St Canice's.

Robin had been moved from Theatre to a single cubicle beside the Ward Station. All the panoply of surgery was there. Jars, tubes, drip-stand. On the bed, he lay inert. A cage distorted the outline of his body.

I left him undisturbed.

Next day I began to realise what major surgery involved in suffering. The loose crumpled Theatre gown, embroidered 'St Canice's', revealed a gauze pad over a dark blood-stained wound. Swollen lips, cracked and encrusted in dried mucous. Pale damp skin; summer's fading freckles livid as a peppering of birth marks. The punctured hand tied to the side rail of the bed; bandaged fingers groping for human contact.

The writhing, gasping, 'Sore! Oh, it's getting sore now!' An in-jection.

His body temperature fluctuated. He felt too hot, then too cold. Only sheets and a coverlet were provided in summertime. The heating system was off. A convector was supplied to counteract the hypo-thermic effect of the blanketless bed. I constantly adjusted and readjusted the controls in an effort to keep him tolerably comfortable.

The tiny room was cluttered with equipment. There was space only for a locker and a straight-backed chair. A wooden crucifix hung above the door. Ceaselessly, the steady whirr of an electric suction machine plugged into a wall socket. After surgery, a narrow plastic Ryle's tube had been inserted down Robin's nose and into the stomach to draw off secretions and gastric juices. It did its job erratically. At regular intervals, a nurse came to disconnect the tube from the glass jar into which it emptied. She attached a syringe and drained off the thick fluid by hand-manipulated suction. Each time, Robin woke from his drugged sleep and whined with pain.

'Stop it! Please stop. I beg you. Stop!' His body revolted. He gagged ineffectually; a dry retching. His stomach was empty of everything except painful sensation.

Progress. One day passed, then another.

He was propped up on pillows and became more lucid, more aware.

'I heard someone say there were twenty stitches. I'm so scared I'll never get out of here.' He gargled with water, a luxury. The residue he spat out into a kidney-shaped dish. His shoulders flopped back against the pillows in exhaustion.

Fear fluttered in his mind. 'I'm afraid to sleep now in case they take me away for another operation. Last time they said it was only for an X-ray, and look what happened to me.'

'Robin, surgury requires a signature of consent for general anaesthesia. We'll never allow any further operations. That's a promise.' I meant it.

The Chaplain called. I wasn't there but Robin talked about it.

'I asked him about God and Heaven. He said that maybe there'll be a great war or a nuclear explosion and everything will end. Then – there will be God! To understand God, he said you could think of a good road marred by accidents. Or a lovely room thick with dust. Or a garden overgrown with weeds. But Heaven is where everything is perfect all the time.'

I nodded, simulating agreement, evicting the query as to why an Omnipotent God had chosen to create an imperfect world.

When the stitches were removed and the pad replaced by a dressing secured by an adhesive strip, I saw the second incision. A red weal, several inches long. Vertical, beside the navel.

Robin began to eat, to move about again. His physical deterioration was apparent. Spindly legs weakly supported his reduced body weight.

His eyes protruded slightly in the gaunt pale face. His hair was thick and shaggy, a knotted tangle over the forehead where restless fingers had twisted it into damp coils.

Two weeks after surgery, Robin was discharged. Mr Verkonnen arranged to see him regularly for check-ups. The prognosis was vague. The beginning of the end would manifest its own symptoms – probably in about three months' time.

The cubicle had to be vacated after lunch. When we arrived to collect him, Robin had been dressed and was perched disconsolately in the Sitting Bay opposite the Station. He was balanced uncomfortably on the edge of a chair. He stood up stifly.

'My trousers hurt my tummy,' he said. We relieved the pressure of the waistband on his abdominal wound and secured his trousers loosely with a safety pin.

He was debilitated and lachrymose. But once home again, he seemed more contented. Bob had repapered and decorated his bedroom. Racing cars roared silently round the walls. It delighted Robin.

Ahead of us stretched the summer that would be his last.

TWO

July

'O child of laughter, I will go
The meadow ways with you, and there
We'll find much brighter stars . . .'
Patrick Kavanagh (*To a Child*)

When time is limited, it becomes infinitely precious. Everything has significance. Everything is memorable.

Hungrily, I watched facial expressions, noticed mannerisms, listened to the range of voice cadences. I stored up memories for a future when only remembrance would remain.

Quickly I realised that Robin was not a convalescent but an invalid. Holy Innocents' had supplied us with a bottle of red medicine to counteract digestive cramps. For abdominal soreness, Codeine tablets were recommended.

His bowel motions were frequent and very loose. Consequently, the area from the buttocks' cleavage to the scrotum was angry and red. He gripped the side of the bath and shuddered as I gently cleansed the raw skin and applied an analgesic cream.

His first night at home was marred by broken sleep. I heard him whimpering, moaning, as he tossed around. Repeatedly I tiptoed to his room, frustrated by my own inability to help. Finally, the futility of it struck us both. I settled him down beside me in my own bed. The relief of having someone with whom to share a wakeful night gradually eased his mind. Eventually he drifted into sleep.

In the darkness, I lay wide-eyed and prayed. 'No prayer goes unheard.' The answer might not be that for which I hoped but, in His wisdom, God knew best. I tried to subjugate my thoughts, my doubts. The traditional prayer formulas escaped me. I improvised . . .

'O God! Wherever or whatever you are, help this tortured weak child whose body is being wracked by daily suffering. Whose mind is becoming haunted by fear of what may lie ahead. Fear is growing in me, too. Just give him this summer free of sadness and then take him quickly. Please, please . . .'

Shallow breathing beside me. A damp hand, fingers locked in mine. Night silence.

Robin's schoolfriends came to see him but he wasn't ready for their boyish exuberance and quickly tired. He stayed most of the day in bed, coming down in the evening to watch television.

One night, *The Old Man and the Sea* was screened. It moved us both to tears. Next day, I bought the book for Robin and inscribed it with some lines from the work of Basil Payne, an Irish poet:

> An old man and a boy,
> A boat,
> A fish . . .
> . . . So ends the tale *The Old Man and the Sea*,
> By Papa Hemingway. Portrayed by Spencer Tracy,
> And watched on telly by my son and me.
> 'Well, son?' I question; then observe his face
> Contorted with old man's anguish, child's dismay.
> For twenty minutes he sobs on my knee
> For fish; man; boy; lost Paradise; him; me.

Our fading Paradise. A Sunday in the garden to escape the bumper-to-bumper traffic on the roads. Sunshine. Robin lopping clumsily after a ball. Panting; easing himself into a deck-chair. Billie dropping down beside him. Five-year-old Helen shouting excitedly, just learning to talk. Michael cooing in his pram, registering a four-month-old's delight in living. Bob reading the golf results in the newspaper.

A picnic tea on the grass. Strawberries and cream.

Shorn daisy heads wilting on the lawn. A soft symphony of movement as the breeze played through the beech tree, copper waving fronds on a blue blue sky.

I sat on, savouring moments that would end with summer.

The weather changed to stormy days with blustery winds. Consciously we capitalised on every opportunity, left nothing until later. Later might never come.

It was a dull afternoon, but when the rain showers had blown over Bob asked, 'Like to go fishing?'

Robin and Billie were elated.

We took the boys up on the hills to a gentle valley where a river meandered slowly, brown and shallow by sandy banks, on its journey to the city and the sea. Dark River of no return.

Unknotting tangled lines. Removing slimy algae. Casting. The engrossment of fishermen contentedly catching nothing. The jargon; lead weights, spinners, split shot, flies and bait. Knots; the half-blood, the double loop. Desultory discussions reflecting total absorption. Tiny midges hovering, whirling in a spindrift beneath the overhanging trees. Tea from a thermos on the riverbank.

Snapshots with a newly purchased camera. A morbid but essential acquisition to capture time on celluloid. We took flash photographs.

A watery sun saluted the end of day. A singsong in the car; Robin's voice was weak in volume but vibrant with happiness . . .

> Will you come with me, a Stóir?
> When the summer day is o'er
> And the rooks are winging homewards in the sky;
> We'll go home thro' Slaney Valley
> You and I . . .

Intermittent pain had become part of life now. It started after meals. We combated it with the prescribed medicine.

The day following the fishing trip, medication brought only brief relief. By teatime, it had developed to severe cramps. Robin struggled to distract himself. He stuck pictures in a scrap album, read a *Swallows and Amazons* adventure. Bob moved the television set to Robin's bedroom.

But the pain persisted. It grew in strength until his screaming could be heard on the street outside. I telephoned the doctor. Robin tossed and rolled on the bed. Gripped the pillowcase in clenched teeth. Grasped his abdomen. Doubled up his legs in an attempt to alleviate the pain.

The GP came and examined him. Then he drove away to his surgery and returned with morphine. It was 10.30 p.m. before Robin dropped into an induced sleep. The doctor sat by his bedside, voice professionally soft and soothing, waiting for the injection to take effect.

'If you've any trouble during the night, be sure to call me,' he said.

At midnight, we had to telephone again. He came.

Six hours later, another phone call. He gave Robin a third injection. 'I'll ring Holy Innocents'. Mr Verkonnen will have to see him.'

Later I telephoned the hospital to confirm the booking. The receiver was clammy in my hand.

'Yes, Mrs Heron,' Admission Sister's voice was pleasant, efficient. 'Your doctor has been in touch with us. It would be best if you brought Robin over as soon as possible.'

Ten days had passed since his discharge.

His summer was over.

THREE

July, August, September

'Man's body is so small, his strength of
suffering so immense.'
Rabindranath Tagore

Formalities were quickly dispensed with at Holy Innocents'. Admission Sister didn't offer us the anaesthetic authorisation form for signature and I was relieved at her omission. It saved explanations, for I was determined not to sign it. Robin trusted my word. I had promised there would be no further surgery. There would be none.

Sister arranged for a return to St Canice's Ward. 'He knows the staff there. It will be familiar to him.'

It was familiar. And terrifying.

Bob carried Robin, swathed in blankets, to the cubicle which he had vacated less than a fortnight before. He laid him on the bed.

A House Surgeon came to examine him. It was an impossible task. The houseman called for assistance. Two doctors and three nurses held Robin down while he struggled and hollered and screamed. The tiny room was a scrummage of white figures, threshing limbs, threats and exhortations. Finally, he was subdued. From the Sitting Bay, I watched the whole monstrous pantomime.

An X-ray was arranged. We went over the landing to Radiography. Bob eased Robin into a chair and we queued up. A confused threesome in the Waiting Room. A nurse was sitting there too, a slip of paper in her hand, lost in her own private world.

Without warning, Robin vomited over the floor. Splatters of partially digested food dribbled on his dressing-gown. I tried ineffectively to clean up the mess with tissues.

A girl in an all-enveloping apron commuted between the Waiting Room and the Radiography Unit. Apologetically, she explained that the staff were at their coffee break.

The time seemed interminable but eventually they returned.

Back at St Canice's, Robin lay moaning on the bed. I watched the Ward Station. Presently the X-rays were delivered: incomprehensible studies in light and shade. The plates were clipped to a viewing box, then illuminated. The housemen and Sr White studied them.

My nerves were screaming. I walked the corridor; sat down in the Sitting Bay; paced the passage again.

Oriel Verkonnen appeared. He was dressed for surgery: little green cap, shapeless green gown tied at the waist, mini gumboots. Presumably he had seen the X-rays, been briefed by his House Surgeons, for – having looked in on Robin – he came out to talk with me.

He explained that there appeared to be an obstruction in the intestines. Maybe only a twist, but he would have to operate again immediately.

I was incredulous. 'But if it's hopeless, Mr Verkonnen, why?'

He didn't waste words. 'It may be something minor. We can't leave him in this pain.'

I was desperate. Robin had trusted me. I had assured him that there would be no further surgery. I struggled to explain.

'I promised him there'd be no more operations. I promised him, and he believed it, and I meant it.'

Mr Verkonnen volunteered to tell Robin.

'It's not a case of who is to tell him, Mr Verkonnen. It's surgery itself that's the problem . . .'

But he moved away and went into the cubicle. I hovered near the door.

'Robin, I have to do a small operation,' he said.

Terror struck with cyclonic force. Robin screamed, almost hurling himself off the bed. A posse of medical staff appeared. Robin lashed out at them, finger nails tearing at the restraining hands which tried to hold him down.

A screaming, snarling, trapped wild thing; clawing, scratching, biting.

Forcibly he was pinned down and given an injection.

He was lifted on to a mobile stretcher. A Theatre Orderly, with a mask pushed up over his forehead, comforted him as he wheeled him along. I walked beside the trolley through the double swing doors and into the Theatre concourse. Silent tears streamed down my face.

Robin noticed my distress. 'Don't cry, Mum. Don't cry.'

The trolley was parked to one side while another patient was rolled away – an inert childish figure, accompanied by a nurse pushing a drip-stand.

Robin was relaxing now, the injection taking effect. 'Will you wait, Mum? Will you be here all the time?'

Theatre Sister came over and took my place beside him. She had been on duty since early morning and looked tired, but her voice was patient and gentle. 'Don't worry, Mrs Heron.'

She told me how long he was likely to be, but nothing registered in my brain: nothing.

I squeezed Robin's hand. To kiss him was too final. Something of my own terror might communicate itself to him.

Sister shepherded me out of the Theatre precincts. Calmly now. Keep calm. I walked in a daze. There must be no histrionics. Easy does it. Keep calm.

. . . I remembered the death of Melody, the old mongrel collie who had been part of my childhood. A fluffy cuddlesome puppy salvaged from the Stray Dog's Home.

The veterinary surgeon had laid him flat on the surgical table and expertly slipped a muzzle over the unprotesting head. He had snipped a patch of brown hair from the foreleg and filled a hypodermic syringe.

'Just talk to him quietly now. Don't excite him.'

I had fondled the gentle head. 'There, Melody. There, there. That's the good boy.'

There was a reflex jerk as the needle penetrated the skin. The syringe emptied so slowly, slowly. The occasional convulsive shudder. It emptied lethally.

And I had stood by the greying diseased muzzle and gently stroked the silky head, quietly repeating his name again and again. Limpid brown eyes held mine trustfully and I murmured reassurance. On and on – until the breathing stopped. And only a still dead thing remained on the formica-topped table . . .

In the car, I talked incessantly. Bob understood that I had to burn up the powderkeg of hypertension. He let me rant on, uninterrupted.

'I hope he dies. I just hope he dies right there on the table. Apart from the shock to the surgeon and the anaesthetist, it would be the best thing. That way he'll cheat further pain. I hope he's dead right now!'

* * *

Robin was just surfacing from anaesthesia when we returned. His skin was translucent and deathly pale. A pretty nurse with a Victorian-cameo face sat by his bed. She supported his hand on her knee. A plastic identification bracelet had been sealed to his arm. Gently she laid his hand on the sheet.

'His wrist had been tied to the bed to prevent him pulling out the drip,' she explained. 'But I know him from the last time he was here. He's a sensible little boy so I removed the strapping. It leaves him more comfortable.'

She left us alone with him for a few minutes. His pallor was ghastly. His eyelids flickered in half-recognition.

'Mum! Oh Mum! I'm panicking. And you look so tired . . .'

His mind began to wander. 'The old man in the boat. The fish. That film . . . But my rod is safe. Daddy'll keep my rod safe.' He drifted into temporary oblivion.

His shallow breathing punctuated the silence. This time, there was no suction draining machine; only a drip-stand.

A transistor was playing in the Sitting Bay. A child turned up the volume. 'Here comes Summer' – a band introduced the signature tune. The music faded down for the presenter's voice-over. Upped again and died away. The interviewer ad-libbed – 'and today we're at Carrig-namara, where the Shannon River meets the sea. So let's talk to some of the happy holidaymakers enjoying themselves this sunny after-noon . . .'

Innocuous chatter. Wish-you-were-here messages for the folks back home. Musical interludes.

Life was going on. Was reality there, with the carefree crowds? Was reality here, in the tormented body of a child, ambushed by tribes of cells alienated from their healthy neighbours, creeping insidiously on in a dance defeated only by death?

'Oh God! I'm so sick of it all. So weary. So frightened.' My voice had echoed my thoughts aloud. In prayer? In despair? I no longer knew.

Bob put his arm around my shoulders and held me.

Mr Verkonnen's secretary phoned St Canice's Ward. The surgeon wanted to see us. We traipsed the familiar passages, through the Coffee Bar, and into the warren of rooms and surgeries of the consultants' clinic.

We were ushered into Mr Verkonnen's office. He was sitting at his desk and rose to meet us. We sat down on straight-backed chairs. He dispensed with introductory comments.

Robin's condition was hopeless, he told us.

'I'm very sorry,' he added. There was a pause. His head dropped on to his hands. I noticed his hands; small neat hands with square-tipped fingers. Child surgery is delicate; fine, artistic in its own genre.

I was stunned. Where was the three months' remission? The summer of borrowed time? Where had it gone? I had to know, to be sure I understood him correctly.

'You mean – you don't mean that Robin's going to die? To die now?'

Through the catatonic barrier of stupor I heard his reply. Robin would last only a few days. From the rate of development since the last operation, it would probably be less than a week. Again he paused; then added that Robin had nearly died during the operation that morning.

Mother of God! Less than a week! But maybe it would be a week of post-surgical agony.

My voice was a whisper. 'How will he die?'

He explained that often there was a coma; an easing away so that one hardly knew it had happened.

Another pause. Mr Verkonnen brushed back the white-blond hair that had fallen over his forehead. 'This is dreadful for you. Dreadful,' he said simply.

Bob broke in, quietly. 'There is one thing, Mr Verkonnen. The visiting hours. We'd like to be with Robin as much as possible but we've a four-month-old baby. Could you possibly arrange for us to be admitted a little later in the evenings? You see, we sometimes find it very hard to be here before eight.'

Mr Verkonnen replied that since it was only for a short time, we might be able to adjust our domestic schedules to fit in with hospital regulations.

I felt chilled by the tone. But my flagellated spirit stirred. Authority could be circumvented by strategy. However, right now there was the variance between the prognosis and the reality to be explained.

I probed. 'What did you find when you operated?'

Mr Verkonnen's soft voice dropped. There was a growth, he said.

'And did you remove it?'

He answered succinctly that a surgeon must make his own decisions.

It was familiar in layman's language. 'All they could do was sew him up.' The crashed car, the wrecked aircraft, the obsolete battleship. All fated for the breakers' yard.

The interview was over.

Robin was a write-off.

Static crackled in my brain as we pulled in to the car park that night. I was no fighter enjoying the parry and thrust of abrasive verbal encounters. Always I had adopted evasive strategy; anticipated confrontation and avoided it by placation or subservience. I never ventured consciously on a collision course, for inevitably it meant defeat for me. Faced with resistance, I invariably capitulated.

It was a wisdom born in the isolated world of an only child. I had developed an awareness of duty. Decisions were made for me and in consultation with me. I never questioned the voice of Authority, never queried its credentials or logic. My anxiety to please always eroded my courage.

Now, for the first time in my life, I had to take a stand. At least cowardice had taught me tactical cunning.

It was 8.30 p.m. Visiting hours were over. The Night Porter glanced up as we pushed open the door. I was expecting a difficult confrontation, so I spoke decisively. 'Our son is a patient in St Canice's,' I said pleasantly. 'He's very ill and we've permission to see him at any time.' I checked the impulse to elaborate any further.

He accepted my explanation and expressed his regrets. An *entente cordiale* was established.

It was a salutary victory. But anticipation of a fray had drained my waning vitality, and wearily I found my way to St Canice's Ward.

A 'Special' had been called in to sit with Robin. She was an Agency Nurse, supplementing the regular Holy Innocents' night staff. A brooch on her lapel identified her. 'Nurse O'Neill'. She left us with him.

Robin was sleeping. He wore no clothes. His skin was tinctured with a green hue from the faint wattage of the night-light. The bulb had a death-reflecting glow. The refracted glimmer from the green painted walls illuminated the cubicle eerily.

On the bedside locker, beside the blood-pressure testing case, was a clipboard of copious leaflets. Discreetly, I eased the cubicle curtains together so that I could pry unobserved. Principles and integrity were sabotaged by necessity.

I leafed through the notes and found a report. Isolated phrases of technical jargon. Facts, ball-pointed on to paper. I jotted them down on a cigarette packet '. . . massive growth on back abdominal wall . . .'

So there was more than a blockage in the intestine! But had the 'massive growth' been removed? There was no one to ask. No one prepared to answer.

Hastily I replaced the file as Nurse O'Neill came in. With contrived casualness, she picked up the clipboard and took it away to the Ward Station.

Twice in one evening, I had contravened the code of rules and twice escaped castigation. The seeds of courage, conceived in desperation, started to bud.

I left the sunshine outside and climbed the stairs to St Canice's. A cheerful Danny whirled by in his wheelchair. The influx of Saturday visitors made it an exciting day for him.

The tiny face of Cathal peered down the stairwell. A smile of recognition touched his features; then vanished. I was no longer part of his world. Just a half-remembered person that used to visit the boy who had once shared his room. Paths briefly touching, then diverting. He continued his vigil; waited for his faithful 'family' who would not shatter his illusion of security.

Overnight I had pondered and eschewed the limited facts as I knew them.

Robin was dying. He had a massive growth. It would bring pressure on his bladder, bowels, liver, internal organs; on everything intrinsic to the maintenance of life itself. When the system could fight no longer, life would cease.

An intraveneous drip fed into his body. I read the label on the up-turned bottle which drained steadily into the vein. 'Saline' – it meant nothing to me. If it were sustenance, wouldn't its removal expedite the inevitable end? Robin was destined to die soon anyway. The virulence and rapidity of the growth ensured that; a process which might become increasingly painful as the body was forced to a halt.

The Right to Live – the Right to Die? Robin's position was hopeless. So why the IV drip? Why, why why?

In the passage, I met the hirsute houseman with the desert boots. I questioned him.

He explained. 'The drip which you see is just saline. A salty solution administered as a transfusion to prevent dehydration. It makes it easier for the body to absorb drugs.'

I persisted. 'Will he need drugs, then? Will there be pain?' It was a plea for communication. It ignited no response.

I continued. 'Mr Verkonnen said he had found a "massive growth" . . .'

'I know. I was in Theatre. It's a lymphosarcoma.'

'What did Mr Verkonnen do, doctor? Remove it all, or is it still there?'

There was a pungency in his tone. He replied but did not answer. 'How familiar are you with Histology, Mrs Heron?'

I admitted defeat. 'I don't even know what the word means.'

Perfunctorily, he had extricated himself from the inquisition.

Back in the Sitting Bay, I flopped into a chair. A small boy, physically disabled, trundled by in a strange contraption – a wooden box, mounted on four wheels, low to the ground. It was painted a gay green, with white bunny rabbits flirting amongst flowers. A woman watched him with bovine interest. I looked at them both hypnotically. A fulgurant flash seared through my mind.

Frantically I had beamed out SOS signals for any explanation which would clarify the composite queries that beleaguered my brain. I had maintained a controlled calm, had given no display of histrionics through the traumatic weeks. But there had been no recognition of my need. My mandate now was to delve into technical fields and assimilate the relevant facts about cancer. Anything to clear my confusion.

Nathan. I thought of him suddenly. Nathan would help me. Nathan – ex-Roman Catholic priest. Medical doctor. Friend, confidant, mentor.

Nathan did help. Right to the end.

*　　　*　　　*

Robin vomited several times next day. No sooner had he settled into sleep than he was woken for a blood pressure check. The inflatable rubber band was wound round his upper arm, the cuff pumped up, the pressure on the artery beneath registered on the manometer; and a notation made on his chart.

It was a simple two-minute procedure but it left him miserable and restless each time. Drawing on embryonic courage, I suggested to Sr White that as Robin's death was a foregone conclusion, this routine could be dispensed with. Logic, fortified by tenacity, won the round. The instrument was removed. If the checks were continued, at least he was not disturbed when we were there. Every modicum of discomfort spared him was a salve to my spirit too.

Night-time brought a new problem. Nurse O'Neill appeared on the passage; a trim figure in a trouser suit, carrying a hold-all.

Robin spotted her. 'Not her! Please don't leave me with her. She wanders off during the night and closes the door so that I won't disturb the others.'

There were no bells. Unless the cubicle door was left open, a child could scarcely be heard if he called out.

I tried to reason with him. 'A junior nurse is also on Ward duty all night, Robin.'

'I know. But it's Nurse O'Neill who's with me. And she frightens me. Last night she said I'd no manners. And when I tried to turn over on my side for an injection, she kept saying "Hurry up, there! Hurry up!"'

Out to the Station. God! I'm going to gain a reputation as a virago! I explained Robin's distress to Sr White who was just going off duty.

She was sympathetic. 'Nurse O'Neill is an Agency Nurse. We call on them for special cases when we're short-staffed. Sometimes they're not used to children. I'll see what we can do.'

I returned to Robin. He watched the passage. Nurse O'Neill, neatly uniformed now, checked in at the Station. There was a conversation. Faces turned towards Robin's room. I sat by his bedside, talking sporadically; anything to distract him. Anything to brace myself for trouble if it came.

Nurse O'Neill pushed open the cubicle door. Robin turned his face away. Great watering eyes flooded with unshed tears.

She opened fire at once. It was directed at him. 'I hear you don't like me, Robin.'

His mouth trembled. I sat silent, moral cowardice enveloping me like a shroud of defeat.

She persisted, a coaxing smile lighting her face. 'Why is that, now? You know I've always been nice to you.'

Uniform gave her the advantage of authority. She stood; I sat. The castigator and the culprit. The inquisitor and the captive. Between us was the child with the quivering mouth under sentence of death.

Weakly I pleaded. 'Please, please let's not go into that now.'

She put down her bag and prepared to stay. Robin caught my hand. The tears spilled down his cheeks. *God! He's not going to live. Can't You let him die in peace.*

God wasn't tuned to my wave-length.

The silence deepened, strengthening her position.

She turned her attention to me. 'I've a child myself, you know . . .' Woman to woman. An appeal to maternal affinity but it struck no chord of identity. One couldn't play games of compromise with a dying child's fear. I stood up.

She continued. 'There's no reason for this dislike, I assure you, Mrs Heron. None at all. I just can't understand it.'

The assertion, in contradiction of Robin's claim, galvanised me into action. 'Please, we won't discuss it here. Or now.'

In agitation, I pushed open the cubicle door, almost tripping over her hold-all. I blundered my way to the Station where curious eyes had been watching the confrontation.

Decisive and positive action paid dividends. Sr White responded promptly.

Following a few internal phone calls, a gentle elderly nurse was transferred from duty with the infants in Cherubims' Ward. She would do vigil with Robin that night.

Early next morning, Holy Innocents' telephoned.

'Robin is in severe pain. Short of brute force, it's impossible to give him an alleviating injection. Would it take you long to come over?'

I threw on my clothes and arrived breathless fifteen minutes later.

As I ran along the ward passage, I heard his screams. A phalange of nurses surrounded him with compassionate concern. He flung himself across the bed in a frenzy. Quelling my own distress, I took his hand. Tried to introduce a soporific calm into my voice.

His terror was centered on the syringe. Repeated injections were causing hypersensitivity in his buttocks.

Sr White tapped the phial of morphine and broke the seal. She filled the plastic tube. 'Now, Robin, your mother's here. Try to relax and count to ten. Then it will be all over.'

He twisted his face into tight creases. Together we counted. 'One . . . two . . . three . . .'

A gentle knocking on the cubicle door. A nurse looked up. She went out. 'Six . . . seven . . .'

'The Chaplain would like to see you,' she murmured to me.

Still holding Robin's hand, I glanced up. A cassock-clad black figure beckoned me. I asked the nurse to explain Robin's predicament, that right now I must stay with him.

She returned with the renewed request. 'It will only take a moment, Father says.'

Inherent respect for clerical authority, imbibed from home environment and convent education, almost made me waver. My indecision communicated itself to Robin. His bony fingers tightened desperately on mine.

The knocking was repeated. A kefuffle on the passage outside.

'Father says he won't delay you,' the nurse lowered her voice. 'It's about the Sacrament of the Sick . . .'

The Sacrament of the Sick. Extreme Unction. The Sacrament of the Dying. Fire Insurance Policy; arrears of premiums paid up to date in a lump sum. The final shriving of the soul before death. Confess, cleanse and cheat Hell's fires. Last Rites; the paraphernalia; black robe, white lace, purple stole, oil and curcifix. The rituals; the anointing of the sources of sin – the eyes, the mouth, the hands and feet. The awful irony that the senses – seeing, hearing, touching – transmitters of beauty to the spirit, should be regarded as sinful. The confessed evils of a child. The absolution; words of penance. Reception of the Body of Christ. The wafer of bread. Low voices, prayerful intonation . . .

A curd of nausea forced its way protestingly up from my stomach. I trembled in fear and apprehension. In the realisation that here, against the influential power of a great historic church, I must now take another stand.

My decision was made. I turned to the waiting nurse.

'Please tell Father that I cannot leave Robin now. Tell him I respect his dedication and ask him to appreciate my feelings too.'

The trembling continued as I sat down for the start of my four-hour session with Robin.

The morphine began to take effect. His pain gradually abated. Sr White sensed the strain. She brought me a cup of tea. The nausea subsided. Her kindness made me cry.

Since Robin's life was now counted in days, we worked a shift rota. Bob, myself and my mother relieved each other by his bedside. It was a fourteen-hour day, ending about an hour before midnight. He had a dread of being left alone. Since the comfort of our company was all we could give him, somehow we adjusted our domestic life to his needs. Friends rallied round with practical help.

Bob was sitting with Robin when the Chaplain returned in the afternoon. The priest explained the form of the Sacrament of the Sick. The soothing effect it had on the spirit, the physical improvement which often showed in the body.

Bob played for time. 'I'll discuss it with my wife, Father,'

Later we talked it over and together we decided against it.

'Robin is sinless,' I declared firmly, then added, 'even if one did believe in the concept of sin.'

Bob looked at me quizzically. He explained his reasoning. 'I feel that God would not judge him harshly even if he had transgressed.'

From differing viewpoints, we had arrived at the same conclusion. Robin must be left in peace. He had developed a suspicion of everyone and everything unfamiliar. No further intrusion must be allowed to trouble his mind.

Because I was too malleable in discussion, I decided to write my explanation to the Chaplain. It would obviate the danger of being steamrollered into agreement by clever rhetoric.

In writing, I began to recognise the metamorphosis that was taking place in myself – had been taking place over the years. The superfluous branches of religious observance were being lopped off. The bole of faith remained standing upright, but the roots were rotting. Since I didn't require casuistical help, I short-circuited an analysis of my own flummoxed Catholicism, as I wrote my explanation.

Dear Father ———,

By dedication and vocation you are a spiritual healer. Robin, by his birthright, has the subconscious conviction that life will be his. And so indeed it should have been.

What has happened to him is, perhaps, part of a Greater Design which, at this moment, I cannot understand. It is not as I would have planned it for him. Better to have lived and experienced all that life inevitably would have brought; its sadness and happiness. By experiencing these, he would have matured into a full rich human being; an adult with a sensitivity and compassion for all living things; with respect for all men, and a tolerance for those who differed from him in beliefs and attitudes. A man true to his own personal definition of integrity.

But such is not to be.

The suffering Christ promised Dismas: 'This day you will be with me in Paradise.' So it will be for this Chosen Child of ours. Without fear, he will migrate to find his eternal rest.

Yours etc . . .

A note of reply was left at the Station. Sr White handed it to me.

The Chaplain wrote with sincerity and sympathy. While his views differed from mine, he expressed himself with kindness – ending with the promise of a special remembrance in his prayers and Masses.

His dignified acceptance of our stand established an amiable truce between us. He had won my respect.

When occasionally he dropped in to see Robin for a friendly word, we met without embarrassment.

I had done what I had to do.

The next day throbbed by in an increasing volume of pain. There was no pattern to it. Sometimes it struck several times in a few hours, temporarily relieved by morphine.

The nursing staff struggled to alleviate it. Injection followed injection. Robin became violent, scratching and biting me, slapping my face and thrashing his legs to kick out at me. The nurses, in uneasy sympathy, remonstrated verbally with him. He was deaf to everything. Lost in a black abyss of agony.

'Oh God! God save me. The pain. Oh God! Make me better fast. God! I hate you. I hate you!' Another injection.

He sank into oblivion. Exhausted, I threw a pillow on the floor and sat down on it, resting my head on the seat of the chair. I was indifferent to others' opinions; the time for conforming to convention was gone.

Even in his sleep, Robin moaned. Each exhalation of breath was a troubled whimper.

Home life was splintered into fragments. We dished up and gulped down meals, tackled domestic chaos. We couldn't allow ourselves the luxury of leaving the telephone off its cradle. It was imperative that the hospital could establish contact with us at any time.

I tried desperately to keep calm. It was difficult. Organisation was my way of life. It avoided the tensions which, for me, thrived on disorder. Years before I had disciplined my mind against worry over events which I could not control; events which, anyway, frequently did not materialise. Worry was an erosive factor. Abortive to mental serenity, abortive to achievement. Systematically, I reduced stress and anxiety-depression. I had prayed and aligned God to my side, in various causes, in humble supplication. I had always left the future to unravel itself through His will.

Now suddenly everything was crumbling.

But there were things to be done.

I made a courtesy phone call to the Sacred Heart College where Robin had been a pupil and told them of his fate.

Next, I visited the florists'. I explained that my son would be dead before the week had passed. I selected a floral spray from their sample range; carnations and fern. Wrote a card . . . 'Robin, with all our love and memories of happy days'. I was given a receipt.

At home, I checked the notches on the kitchen wall, the pencilled recordings of the childrens' growth rate. The reading was up-to-date. 'Robin. 4 feet 6 inches.'

Then I dialled the undertaker's number and waited for him personally to take the call. His voice sounded familiar over the decades of years since we had met. The idol of the tennis club hops. Popular, yet a basic niceness always emanated from him. I felt he would understand our situation.

Introductions. Explanations. He was solicitous and sounded concerned. I talked on, relieved that his friendliness made the bizarre conversation seem so ordinary.

'It's the last thing we can do for Robin. Ever. And so it must be just right. As perfect as we can make it. You do understand?'

A white coffin. No flowers except the posy which would be delivered by the florists'.

Newspaper insertions? 'Yes. I've thought of that.'

I had drafted it with care. In a semantical struggle, I had managed to remove the words 'Remains' and 'Burial'. I dictated it down the line.

'HERON, on ———, at The Holy Innocents' Hospital. Robin (aged 8 years). Eldest child of Bob and Inez Heron. Removal to Church of St Anne, arriving ——— o'clock. Funeral after ——— o'clock Mass of the Angels, to Cnocmore Cemetery.'

'Do you have a family grave?' The undertaker was a pragmatist.

There was an 'Angels' Plot' in most cemeteries. A sad nameless grass tract allocated to the stillborn, the infants who survived birth only a few hours and small babies.

'Yes. We have a family grave. Only two internments as yet. It's a double plot.'

A family grave; three down, two across. Final earthly resting place in a valley in the hills. A blanket of white marble chippings. Granite headstone rising like an island etched with names and dates. My grandmother and my father were buried there. Old old lady; elderly man; little boy.

Next I collected Robin's school uniform. For him, there would be no shroud of death. I packed the clothes in a small attaché case; then ambiguously labelled it. 'Robin Heron. St Canice's Ward. For Emergency use'.

Sr White deferred to my request.

I left the case beneath the desk in the Ward Station.

An elderly priest called that night.

'I'm Father Sebastian from the Sacred Heart College, Mrs Heron. Actually, I'm librarian in the Junior School. I know Robin well. He's a great reader – very advanced mentally for his age.'

Through the glass door, he looked in on the cubicle. His lips moved in prayer.

'Have you thought of the Sacrament of Confirmation?' he asked. My spirit flinched. Feigning politeness, I explained our reluctance for any ritual that could lead to distress. He understood.

'Might I bring a Relic of the True Cross with which to bless Robin?'

'Well,' I hesitated, 'well, if you think you can do it unobtrusively . . .'

'I will. Of course, I will.'

His gentleness allayed my fears. Then he mentioned that if we were willing, he would like to organise a Guard of Honour of boys from the school to attend the funeral.

When he was gone, I realised that all was done.

I sat down, my mind numbed to a curious state of tranquillity. An unreal calm.

A bright freckle-faced boy, stilled forever in a small white coffin. A phalanx of blazer-clad youngsters, reluctantly recruited to Mass on a day of their summer holidays.

Burial. A name on a tombstone.

Then nothing would remain but memory.

Robin did not die that week. Emaciated but still living, he held on.

The hours by his bedside merged into days. Yet the time didn't seem excessively long to me. I read copiously. I explored a world to which before I had only had a cursory introduction; a new realm of evolution, anthropology and genetics; of philosophy and poetry. All in a struggle to find an answer to the enigma of an omnipotent omniscient Deity who had created such an imperfect universe.

Pain, injections, sleep. Restless reawakening to a further baptism of pain. Christian theology of Baptism; by water, or desire, or blood. *Why, God, why?*

Ward Round. Mr Verkonnen looked in. I waited outside the cubicle door and waylaid him.

'Well, what do you think?'

I still accepted the professional prognosis. The aura of mystique surrounding a consultant created a trust *per se* in all medical personnel.

'I'm worried about him. He's very low,' he replied, moving on. He gave instructions to Sr White.

The pain cycle re-erupted. Delirious and violent, Robin scratched my face as I counted numbers, averting the moment when he must steel himself for the jab of the injecting needle. He kicked and struck at the restraining hands. I put a pile of books within his reach. Paperbacked theology hurtled to the floor as he released the pent-up tension and terror that strangled him.

Gradually the fluid took effect. When he was drowsy, the drip was removed from the vein. The empty stand stood sentinel in the corner.

I looked at him. Bloated hand, swollen from intraveneous seepage. Blood-encrusted nails. The fingers, like tremulous birds, fluttered across the body, scratching the skin. Limbs splayed on the white sheet like the grotesquely twisted corpses in the snows of wartime Leningrad.

From the Sitting Bay, Dietrich's voice drifted. 'Where have all the flowers gone? Gone to pastures every one . . .'

I felt overwhelmed by timeless sadness.

A dull damp evening. A flock of Arctic terns had settled on the hospital lawn, facing into the wind. They rose in desultory flight.

There was a rustle of swishing skirts and the jingle of keys; Sr Regina Rosario came on her rounds. She was Night Sister in charge of Holy Innocents'. Several hundred patients; several hundred charts. Treatment and surgery; observation and aftercare.

The screech of car-brakes; the thud of impact.

The boiling kettle; the blistered skin.

The jar of coloured capsules; the toxaemic stomach.

A rush to hospital for emergency treatment or surgery. Night would bring its tragedies and its triumphs. All was in her custody.

Anonymous on the outsize janitor's keyring which hung from her waist, was the key of the Dangerous Drugs cupboard. Morphine; pethadine; palliatives for pain. But any emergency that demanded her personal attention inevitably meant delay before that key could be released to a qualified duty nurse and the alleviating drug administered to Robin.

I liked Sr Regina Rosario; but with the reservations I unwillingly felt for all Religious. Through opting out of life to serve God in their own way, they alienated themselves from the mainstream of human emotions, frailties and relationships. So it had always seemed to me. But, allowing for the barrier of her vocation, I liked her.

She looked in on Robin.

'Poor little fellow. He's very low. I've been off-duty for a couple of nights and, to me, there's been quite a deterioration since I last saw him.'

The sympathy in her voice made me feel that she really did care.

And desperately I needed someone to care. To care in the long hours of the night when we were gone; when the clock suspended from the ceiling outside the cubicle ticked each slow second away. To care when the pain mounted and drove Robin to screaming dementia. To care enough to telephone us and let us come and sit with him when the faintly glimmering light of his life began to flicker out.

I tried to express my appreciation. It sounded fulsome.

'This is your home. Your convent, Sister. And yet you open your doors to all those who need you . . .'

She looked away from me to Robin. 'While they are in our care, they are our children,' she said simply.

I wrote a letter.

My dear Nathan,

Once, when you showed me a seascape you had painted, I touched your face with my fingers. Spontaneously. An involuntary breaking free from conditioned reticence. And you knew what I felt. You are someone whom it is very easy to love.

We know, you and I, though the words are unspoken – our feelings run deep and so I turn to you. You know me better perhaps than anyone else has ever done. Possibly than anyone ever shall.

So take my hand in yours and wander with me in spirit. I am losing my way in the labyrinth of my own mind. A vagrant in a limbo land that seems to show no chartered paths. No light. Help me . . .

Nathan. We had met by chance many years before. I had driven to the hills above the city at twilight time and sat alone on a stone wall, watching the dying light of day, seeing the kaleidoscope of twinkling colours as the sprawling town turned her night-face to the sky.

A labouring car shattered the stillness. Headlights cut a swathe in the dusk. The driver silenced his engine; switched off the intrusive lights. I heard the metallic clang of a car door. Glancing up, I saw a round-shouldered man, slightly stooped with age, approaching. Under his arm, he carried a sketch-pad.

He leaned against the low stone wall beside me. His voice was little more than a soft whisper. Yet I heard his words.

' "Shall we sit down together for a while?
   Here on the hillside, where we can look down on the city . . .
   Strumpet city in the sunset
   So old, so sick with memories
   Old Mother:
   Some say they are damned . . ." '

I took up the verse.

' "But you, I know, will walk the streets of Paradise
   Head high, and unashamed." '

One of the rarest moments life can give, when strangers share a vision, see with the same eyes.

There was a slow growth of trust, affection, respect; a growth that matured with the passing years.

As a young doctor, fresh from medical school, Nathan enlisted for service on the battle fields of Europe. World War I was dragging ingloriously to its close.

'In the mud and squalor of the trenches, I found God,' he said one evening. We were sitting by his flickering coal fire. 'In the trenches, where other men lost God, I found Him. It didn't give me happiness. For me, it meant total commitment. I didn't want that.'

Being Nathan, he gave everything. After ordination as a Roman Catholic priest, he went to South America. There were many gaps in his life; many breaks in the storyline that told more eloquently than words of an inner conflict.

When I met him, he no longer wore clerical clothes or actively worked the Ministry of Christ. If he offered Mass, it must have been privately. He was attached to no diocese. If he had been laicised, he never referred to it. He appeared to have no ties, no family. Although he didn't practise medicine, he kept himself up-to-date with its advances.

His home was a small self-contained flatlet. The walls of his sitting-room were lined with books. Medicine; theology and philosophy; painting and poetry. Painting was his pastime. Gentle pastoral panoramas and softly muted seascapes.

He was a man at peace with himself and it emanated from him.

Once I had commented on it. 'You're a very restful person to be with, Nathan.' He lifted down a book and handed it to me. Carl Jung's *Memories, Dreams, Reflections*.

'Take it, Inez. It's a very wise book,' he said, resettling himself in his shabby comfortable chair. 'You know, Jung once wrote: "A man who has not passed through the inferno of his passions has never overcome them." ' I leafed through the pages.

Somewhere in those silent decades to which he never referred, he had found his catalyst. His personal crises were behind him now; laid to rest.

I continued my letter to him:

. . . Mine hasn't been a deliberate rejection of Catholicity. It's been a gradual erosion of belief. First, in the Church. Then in the deity of Christ. Now, it seems I'm doubting God himself; his existence.

Many years ago, I turned a myopic eye to those dogmas of faith which, as Catholics, we were bound to accept.

It was unimportant to me that the ovary of Anne, fertilised by Joachim, developed into the foetal Mary – and was immaculately preserved from sin. The Church proclaimed it a Dogma. We must believe in The Immaculate Conception. All right! it didn't matter. Her dead body had been physically assumed into Heaven; a pious tradition, recently become another Dogma of faith by papal pronouncement *ex cathedra*. But such Dogmas didn't trouble me. The atrocities perpetuated by fanatics in Christ's name spilled over from the Crusades, through the Middle Ages, on into the witch hunts of the 19th century. I rejected Christ's Christian Church. But I believed in Christ as God.

From pre-history, man needed God. Voltaire synthesised it: 'If

God did not exist, it would be necessary to invent him.' Man required some Being to ease his mental anguish. To sustain him against the vulnerability of himself to Earth and the elements.

Sun gods. Rain gods. A plethora of Greek and Roman gods. Then the Messiah; long-awaited saviour of Judaism.

Yeshua Bar Joseph. Nazarene carpenter from Galilee. He filled the need at his moment in history. Prophets and seers had foretold His Coming. He gathered his followers and inspired them with His own beliefs. His promise of a brighter future in another world.

Strengthened by martyrdom, His message spread to become a religion of hope for an eternity of bliss. It splintered into sects. Gave birth to *ad hoc* theological experts bent on proving the validity of their own claims to absolute truth.

Religions. Pop-cults. Each century spawned its own interpretation of Christianity. The Roman Catholic Church grew strong in wealth and power. Purged the cultures it touched in a torrent of blood and physical suffering. Killed the unbelievers and the heretics. Silenced the doubters by guarantees of timeless tortures of Hell fires. Yet science, communications and education strengthened the case for the unbelievers.

The Second Vatican Council threw orthodox Catholicity into a ferment. The Irish Catholic Church resisted modernisation. Being geographically insular, it could cling more easily to old institutionalised authoritarian forms. But Vatican Two claimed its victims. I am one.

Indoctrinated in youth. Seeing the old 'truths' crumbling. Struggling to surface from a morass of confusion, I lost my identity as a Christian. Began to find it, as a person. Now I am a nomad searching for a meaning to the enigma of life.

For me, the Church can offer no rational answers. Neither can Christ – a man abandoned by his God and left to die in torment. 'Eloi, Eloi, lamma sabacthani?' For me, until lately, there was only God. Now He too is getting lost in the maze. Help me, Nathan . . .

Nathan's reply came by post next day. I recognised the careful ageing script.

. . . For what I am worth to you, I am always here; whenever you want me. You know that.

Yours is the lonely path all thinking men must take.

Personally, I will never leave the Church. Like Hans Kung, I've received too much from 'this community of faith' to leave it, now or ever. But each man must find his own path and yours will not be easy. Mine, faltering and still wavering, follows that of Simon Peter when he said to Christ: 'To whom shall I go?'

For you, it may be different. But never despair. Perhaps you are much nearer to discovery than you know. Remember Oscar Wilde? Poor persecuted humanitarian genius? He wrote: 'Scepticism is the beginning of faith.' I hope it may be so for you.

His letter ended there.

The Judas Day started inauspiciously. It was no different to any other in what was now the pattern of life.

By its close, my God was dead. Unlikely ever to be resurrected.

I made a routine morning telephone call to Holy Innocents' and received a noncommital reply from a junior nurse. 'No change.'

I took a different route to the hospital, driving down streets bordered with ornamental trees. Their summery beauty brought a temporary spiritual balm. Warm sunshine. A family of young starlings tried their wings in uncertain flight; fluffy feathers ruffling in a soft breeze.

During the morning a new House Surgeon looked in on Robin. He expressed concern at the quantity of drugs registered on the chart.

'Is it bad?' I queried.

He scratched his head. 'It's probably part of the trouble, you know. What Robin identifies as pain may possibly be addiction to morphine.'

I tried logic. 'But in his condition, does it matter?'

He rationalised. 'We have to keep something in reserve for the end. The real pain may get worse.'

I used a direct approach. 'Doctor, he's dying anyway. Does it matter if you push him over the top?'

His voice was solemn. 'There are complications with these drugs. They can disturb the mind.'

I knew little of drug addiction. But I was learning fast to recognise evasion.

'It's a question of ethics, isn't it?' I asked.

Again he scratched his head. 'You could say that, I suppose.'

It was decided to give Robin a bed bath. Sr White and a junior nurse appeared with a trolley, laden with sponges, creams, powder and ointments.

'Please let Mummy stay,' Robin pleaded. Humanely, they agreed.

Expertly, the nurse wet her hands in warm water and smeared soap on her palms. She gently massaged his tender skin. Sr White held him, propped half-upright.

I had not seen his body fully exposed for a couple of weeks. The deterioration was horrific. His shoulder-blades, like sharpened knives, seemed ready to pierce the frail film of skin. Each spinal vertebra thrust its bony nodule down the wasted back. Raw red abrasions marked the pelvic pressure. Tortured body of a diminutive Christus, stripped naked for flagellation.

'See if you can get a foam mattress or a pad,' Sr White murmured to her assistant. 'We use them for children who are a long time in bed,' she explained.

With a towel, she patted Robin's body until it was dry.

He lay back, breathing heavily. Thin emaciated limbs. Skeletal fingers. Skin, a limp webbing holding the bones together. Deep hollows drooped from the clavicles. Every rib, a ripple of wave patterns. A concave collapse below the diaphragm. The scalpel appeared to have incised the site of the second surgical wound. A livid red cicatrice marked the spot, neatly sutured with stitches. Eleven in all.

The sheets were changed. A foam pad was placed beneath the torso, insulating the bones from the pressure of the mattress and a draw-sheet was tucked over it. Dressings were applied. Robin's damp hair was brushed back from his pale forehead.

There was a flickering smile. He whispered his thanks, appreciative of their care and the comfort they had brought him. The ghastly ghost-smile wrenched at my heart. *God! Why do You do these things to the creatures You profess to love?*

A nerve on my eyelid fluttered uncontrollably. I tried to still it with my fingers. Robin watched, suspecting tears.

'Are you crying? Please don't cry. I'm more comfy now.' The hand on the bed reached for mine. Tactile affirmation of affection.

Gradually the twitching eyelid steadied, ceased to quiver. Is this the nearest mortal man ever comes to perfect love? A moment when each, seared by his own pain, reaches out to help the other?

Robin dozed. Then slept.

I prayed. *God! Take him now. Right now, before he reawakens to another bout of suffering. Before he notices the awful condition of his own body. Before some inkling of the inevitable future filters through to terrorise his mind.*

The Judas Day was capricious. Clouds: then sunshine and passing showers. Evening crept in under a lowering sky.

Bob was sitting by the bed as I came along the dimly lit passage. I stepped over a hosepipe; an umbilical cord linking the bathroom with the next door cubicle. A teenage girl, back from surgery, lay on a water mattress. A tap spluttered and hissed.

Sensing my presence, Bob looked up. Finger to lips, he crept from the cubicle.

'Just one bout of pain. It took about ten minutes before the injection came,' he added grimly. 'He's been sleeping since then. I'm going to stretch my legs. Okay?'

I took up position by the bed. Robin stirred uneasily and reached out his hand. His grip tightened on mine. His skin was burning hot.

His breathing changed. Became rapid. Then irregular.

'My legs. Oh, my legs. They feel as if they're in my head. All wound round inside it.' His voice was muzzy. Confused. 'Why is this happening . . . if I'm getting better . . . getting better . . .'

I prayed. *God! I recognise your power. I acknowledge the incomprehensible architecture of your plan. If you want me to crawl to you in spirit, I'm doing so. At this moment, I concede your absolute mastery of all things. You struck Robin with a disease that doesn't cripple. It kills. Now take him from our care to yours . . .*

Bob returned.

. . . Love on a winter's night. Mouth to clinging mouth. Tongues searching; deep exploration. Hot bodies twisting; entwining. Laughter. Words – obscenities by day, erotica between the sheets.

The thrust and rhythm. Harmony of motion. Final accelerative spasms. Damp satiated sleep.

Pregnancy.

'You've a baby boy.' Infant to toddler. Schoolboy with his dreams. Wizened monkey man-child dying on a hospital bed . . .

We sat on. Passive participants in the drama of death.

Robin stirred again. His face was tensed. The eyelids, unshuttered, weirdly exposed his yellowed corneas; unseeing eyes. His breath altered; became shallow – quick panting exhalations.

Across the bed, Bob's glance met mine in empathetic recognition of the change. In the subdued glow of the night-light, we seemed to be watching through a bathysphere porthole; trapped in a green sub-aqueous world. Sensing the unseen presence of death creep closer.

An apprehensive chill prickled my skin. Involuntarily, I shivered. Begged for the final surrender.

God! If you want him, take him now. Before there's any more pain or suffering. No more cat and mouse. Please let him die. While we're here. I don't ask for him to live. Only to die . . .

Tears spilled out from my aching eyes and fell on the hand which Robin held. I eased my fingers free and smudged the wet across my face.

Quick panting breaths.

Bob's head was bowed.

God! Don't play with him. Don't prolong that long long journey to finality. Don't make him a pawn in your game of expiation of man's sins. You let Christ die horribly. Wasn't that enough? Is there never enough? LET IT BE NOW . . .

Shallow panting. The dark presence of Death moved closer. The world stood still. Suffering synthesised in a motionless vacuum.

My spirit shouted wordlessly. Ordered the Almighty. *It's in your power. You marked him apart like Cain. NOW TAKE HIM . . .*

The face on the bed contorted. Brows knitted in furrows of fierce concentration. The distressed breathing faltered. Stopped. A stillness deeper than silence. Time ceased to exist.

My ruptured soul quaked in foreboding. I knew this was my Moment of Truth. The timeless vortex of all my yesterdays. The desolation of an eternity of empty tomorrows.

Robin moved. A deep deep sigh.

Icy sweat rose from the chilled pores of my skin. I willed him to let go. To die.

A gasp of inhaled air. A stalling splutter. Then the breathing resumed. Steadied. Became rhythmic. Normal.

The facial muscles relaxed. Robin slept.

In that moment, my God died. As silently, as treacherously as sunlight on a spring day.

Bob looked up. The Dark Angel was gone. My cataleptic body slumped in the chair, trembling with expunged tension. Bob was still looking at me; two people sharing the solitude of the night with a desperately sick child.

A nurse paused at the door. She spoke softly. 'Robin seems to have settled now. We'll phone you if there's any change.'

We left him in her care.

'Would you mind if we visited the Chapel?' Bob asked tentatively, as though afraid to intrude on a cataclysmic experience of which he was half-aware.

'Of course not, if you want to,' I agreed.

We followed the coloured signs down highly-polished passages to a quiet Oratory. A red Sanctuary lamp flickered in the darkness. The lights from the car park threw the altar into bas-relief. I genuflected; traditional posture for adoration of the Real Presence of Christ in the Tabernacle, Prisoner of Love. I knelt down in customary attitude of prayer.

My thoughts were atrophied in my tired and arid brain. My body flagged with weariness and my tattered emotions were spent. I was glad of the reprieve, the time in which no movement, no feeling was demanded of my exhausted body and mind . . .

What had I expected? A searing solar light on my Damascus road to self-destruction? A Sinaitic voice of Guidance? A wafting-down of spiritual manna to my starving soul?

I had woken that morning with a waning faith in God. By nightfall, I had discovered myself to be an agnostic. A secular humanist.

Quietly, strength percolated back into my spirit. No longer could I be fatalistic, accepting the Will of God, dependent on supernatural help to conquer the crisis. Man was the shaper of his destiny. From now on, I must rely on myself: identify each problem as it arose, analyse it, face it, and solve it within the limits of my ability.

I couldn't stop the ebbing of Robin's life. Cancer would do that in its own way; in its own time. But I *could* fight the acceptance of inevitability which coloured others' attitudes towards him.

In the wake of my disillusionment, came a positive force. I would act.

Someone eased open the Chapel door. A nun moved up the aisle and took her assigned place at a *prie-dieu*. I didn't see her face. Only the familiar shapelessness of her habit marked her apart.

She blessed herself. Spiritual communion with a Creator who was dead to me.

In the vacuum left by lost faith, a tiny ugly seed sprang to life. A resentment of all that this nun stood for. Of all the years of adherence to an authoritarian Church; of the troubled crises and doubts which had assailed my mind whenever my intellect queried the inexplicable mysteries that must be accepted as Divinely revealed truths; of the guilt and inhibitions which repressive indoctrination had scarred on my freedom of thoughts and actions. Catholicism would be tattooed forever on my soul, but my intellect and spirit would conquer fear of final retribution.

My God had died. And I was free.

The ugly seed would germinate quietly. It would grow from an embryonic antipathy to smouldering aversion. It was fated to be many years before it died away to apathetic indifference.

But now I was Man. Man was Man. Homo Sapiens. A species of evolutionary development. A living thing of blood and flesh and tissue. Of mind and memory and intellect. I did not need belief in a God to justify my own mortal existence. Sufficient that I was. That I existed. Lived.

We left the nun at her prayers.

The Armageddon of my soul seemed reflected in the thunderous sky, as we drove home. The threatening storm had broken. Savage sheets of rain lashed the windscreen.

Bob reversed the car in to the driveway – ungaraged, ready for any emergency call.

He pulled out the ignition key and turned to me. We could have been lovers, isolated in a private world. But in the lamp-light, his face was strained and abysmally worn. The sadness, the weariness bonded us together.

'You thought he was going to die tonight, didn't you?' he asked.

I nodded. 'I prayed for it. I prayed for him to die.' My voice fractured. 'Oh Bob! What are we reduced to when we can pray for our own child to die?'

'I prayed too . . .'

'. . . and God didn't answer,' I finished it for him.

He looked ahead at nothingness. The rain lashed the street. He seemed to be choosing his words. When he spoke, it was as though he spoke to himself.

'Yes. Tonight when things were bad for Robin, I prayed that it would end. Peacefully. While we were there. And it didn't. God didn't take him.' He paused. 'He didn't take him. But at least He let him fall into a relaxed sleep. He eased things for him. I'm grateful for that.'

I took his hand.

Simon Peter; tested and proven. Iscariot; the betrayer and the betrayed.

'You've a marvellous faith,' I said quietly. 'I envy you.'

Judas also had been one of the Chosen Twelve.

Next morning Robin was better.

'He had a very good night, according to his chart. And, believe it or not, he's eaten breakfast.' Sr White's professional voice was warm with pleasure.

Live life day by day. That way I'd generate strength in the good times to face the future. Treat each crisis as a situation to which a solution must be sought. Today, perhaps, would be one of the good times.

I felt almost jubilant. My mood reflected Robin's.

'Did Sister tell you I'd had breakfast? Soggy old cornflakes and a cup of tea. But it was delicious. Now come on and we'll play soldiers.'

I took the box from his locker. A graceful line of horses. Plastic muscles rippled in harnessed power as they pulled a gun-carriage. Confederates and Yankees; cowboys and Indians.

On his instructions, I arranged them in serried ranks. He dawdled with them for a while, head propped on thin arm. When he tired of it, he lay back.

'You look very pretty, Mum. You wear nice dresses. You know, everyone here is in uniform. All white. It's lovely to see a bit of colour. Will you wear a different dress each time you come in?'

'Of course, if you like.'

He was pleasantly relaxed. 'Now tell me all that's happening at home. Talk to me.'

When I'd exhausted the word pictures, he wanted more. 'Tell me about when you were young.'

I glanced around for inspiration and saw the abandoned soldiers. Then I began to talk of my war-time childhood, of rationing and the blackout, of bicycle transport and searchlights and gas masks. I spoke of Ireland's neutrality and the occasional stick of misplaced bombs.

Presently, he turned to a magazine, and began to read. *Look and Learn.*

The clatter of the trolley sounded from the Ward kitchen. A team of nurses scurried down the passage to take delivery of it. Robin watched its progress from cubicle to cubicle. Plates of steaming stew; scoops of potato and vegetable.

'I'm hungry. Do you think I could have some dinner?'

Sr White compromised and ordered a soft-boiled egg, mashed up in a cup, and a thin wafer of buttered bread. Robin chewed it carefully as instructed, relishing the forgotten flavours. Then he washed it down with tea.

Presently the pain started. He had an injection but it brought no relief. Another followed – a muscle relaxant, the Houseman said. It began to take effect but a new complication arose almost immediately.

Relaxation caused the muscles to slacken, the bowels to open. It had a purgative result. There was no time to run for a bedpan. Robin's penis rose erect in the swollen genitals. An arc of urine sprayed out forming a puddle on the sheet.

He felt the involuntary muscular movement and winced at the bowel contractions which he couldn't control.

'I'm going to dirty the bed. God! I think it's coming. Oh! the pain . . .'

He began to writhe. The veins in his neck throbbed with effort. His face contorted. Back arched. Teeth grinding together.

Brown faeces inched slowly, slowly out into the yellow pool of urine.

I gently wiped excrement from the soiled skin and covered the malodorous heap with tissues.

'There's more. I know there's more. If it's sore like this for hours, I'll yell and yell. I'll just begin to yell.'

Urine pattered like obscene amber rain on the stretched cotton sheet. Stale faeces released their gaseous smell. I tried to breathe through my mouth to avoid retching. But the miasma hung heavy in the air.

Robin's tormented torso arched. His wet feet padded inch by inch across the sheet until he lay sideways on the befouled bed, clear of the mound of crushed tissues.

'I think it's over. The Big Jobs. They shouldn't be so painful, should they? They're not proper and normal. God! It can't get any worse than this.'

I murmured reassurance. 'I'll ask a nurse to change the sheets.'

'No. Not yet. Not now. Just wait till I've rested and the soreness is gone from my bottom.' His arched body flopped down.

Purged by pain, he was now subjected to the final degradation. The indignity of lying, fully conscious, in a cesspool of his own slurry. His body defiled.

Minutes passed. 'I think that's all there is of it. There doesn't seem to be any more coming. Could you call a nurse, please?'

They waived the rules at his request and let me gently wash the flaky skin. Then they changed the sheets and tidied up the bed. A fresh towel was placed under his head to absorb the sweat.

But a new fear began to play on his mind. 'What will I do if this goes on? If every time I'm hungry and eat something – this happens?'

It didn't happen like that.

Sometimes several days passed before his bowels would expel their accumulated load. Nearly always he had sufficient muscular warning to call for help.

A bedpan was slipped under the scrawny bruised buttocks. He was levered up into a half-propped position. I sat behind him on the bed, supporting his shoulders against my body. His fingers, spread-eagled on the mattress, maintained his balance. Up to twenty minutes could elapse before defecation brought relief. Sometimes a nurse, gloved fingers lubricated with antiseptic jelly, inserted a glycerine suppository up the abused anal passage. This invariably brought results, but it also aggravated the mental anxiety for him.

He began to sleep less during the day, to play with toys and to read again. His appetite increased.

The supply from the hospital kitchen only came up at regular meal times. The Ward kitchen carried a small float of basics: eggs, bread, milk, cornflakes. We started to bring in food that suited his whims and complied with his dietary limitations. We did not conceal what we were doing and the authorities did not veto it.

Robin's tastes varied from plain biscuits to cereals and cakes. Inevitably, when his hunger was satisfied, a spasm of pain started. He was trapped in a circle of multiple suffering.

My relationship with Sr White had been positive and progressive. She seemed to appreciate the mantle of calm with which I tried to cloak my reaction to the moments of crisis. And there was the practical asset that, by ministering to Robin's needs ourselves, we released her junior staff for general nursing duties in the Ward.

One day, as I emerged from the cubicle with a laden bedpan discreetly covered in a regulation cloth, she came from her Station.

'I'll take that from you. I just want to check if there's any blood in his motions.'

'Has there been any to date, Sister?'

She nodded. 'Sometimes we've found traces of it.'

'Would it have any significance?'

'Well, it might mean internal haemorrhageing. Something malfunctioning. It's hard to tell.' She took the bedpan. 'Has Mr Verkonnen said anything to you lately?' she asked.

'I hardly ever see him, Sister. Has he discussed Robin with you?'

She hesitated a moment before replying; then, choosing her words with care, said that he wasn't a very communicative man.

I smiled at what, to me, was an understatement.

'Maybe I should make an appointment to see him in his consulting rooms?' I prompted. 'It might give us some idea of what's going on . . .'

'Do that,' she agreed immediately, nodding towards the house phone in the Ward Station.

'Mr Verkonnen won't be in until tomorrow,' his secretary explained down the line.

'Do you think I could get him at home, at this hour?' It was late afternoon.

'Well, I suppose you might. Or you could make an appointment to see him here tomorrow.'

I thanked her, not asking for his home number. Requests could lead to refusals.

My finger traced the column of letters . . . procrastination could be the thief of courage. I found the name, dialled the digits and waited.

Mr Verkonnen's voice came on the line. I introduced myself. I told him of our concern at the evolving pattern of pain from Robin's astricted bowel motions, the increasing intensity of agony from the cancerous growths.

The telephone has potential for breaking the barriers between people. No facial gestures nor visual expressions of impatience can set or shatter the mood of a conversation. It can be a great equaliser. But not this time.

Mr Verkonnen replied politely, and I heard myself prattling on to fill his silent gaps.

'Possibly the bowel pains come from the increasing virulence of the growths?' He agreed it was a possibility.

'Maybe the growths are impeding the discharge of waste matter?' That too was a likelihood.

I asked how long this could continue? Not more than a few weeks, maybe less, he felt.

In a gush of apologies for my intrusion, I said goodbye. My courage had collapsed and I slumped back in the Staff Sister's chair, little more enlightened than before I had dialled and considerably more deflated.

Mr Verkonnen's surgical ability, technical skill and professional prestige positioned him in the ranks of leading eminent surgeons. But, as a communicator, I ranked him almost zero.

The shiny receiver was clouded with a wreath of sweat.

July slipped away into August.

Our friends did not fail us. They were indispensable. They took Billie and Helen out for day trips and invited them to tea. Billie knew that Robin was very sick and must still stay in hospital. He did not question any further.

Each day, a neighbour called and took Michael's carry-cot to her home where she looked after him until late evening. I prepared his feeds, left bottles and nappies ready, and surrendered him to her care. Her own family was adult now, and despite the pressures of irregular mealtimes for them, she coped with Michael too.

Letters came. They reflected the extraordinary simple faith of Irish Catholicism from which I felt alienated. Yet their sincerity was obvious. It touched me.

> How very sorry I am to hear that the Cross has knocked at your door. May Our Lord's Holy Will be done. He knows best, doesn't He? You must trust and pray that Our Lord may give your little boy a longer lease of life if it is for His greater honour and glory . . .

> I am with you in suffering at the thought of your little Angel suffering so much. God knows best. It must be for something big, like the saving of our souls or the salvation of Russia that Robin is the victim. If possible, try and see the silver lining behind the cloud . . .

> You have been specially selected as God's baby-sitters . . .

> You must not pray for Robin's recovery. Instead leave him in God's hands and pray that His Will be done . . .

Holy Pictures came.

Rita: 'Saint of the Impossible'. *Anne and Jude:* joint patrons of 'Hopeless Cases'. *Peregrine:* patron of cancer victims.

There were 'Pious Objects' too.

A loan of Padre Pio's mittens – the stigmatist of San Giovanni Rotondo. The stole-of-office worn by Fr John Sullivan, a Jesuit priest who was respected as a miracle worker. Lourdes water – from the spring where Bernadette Soubirous had scratched the earth at the Grotto, on the instructions of the Immaculate Conception, and brought forth a stream of healing water.

Phone calls were the most gruelling. Our grief was too poignant, too personal, to be discussed with ease. I listened, appreciating the concern of the callers.

'The Age of Miracles hasn't passed.'

'While there's life there's hope.'

'Robin was a good little boy. He'll go straight to Heaven.'

'There's only one thing nicer than having a son on earth, and that's to have a son in Heaven.'

At a bus stop, one evening, I gave a lift to an acquaintance. I was returning from Holy Innocents'. She was en route back from the city, laden shopping bags bulging. She settled herself in the passenger seat and launched into conversation.

'You know, when I tell my friends about Robin, I always say it's just terrible. I say it's so awful that such a tragedy should happen to such nice people. But you'll get great blessings out of this. Wait and see . . .'

I was stunned into speechlessness. She couldn't really be chattering so insensitively. But she was.

'Maybe your little girl – Helen isn't it? – well, maybe she'll improve mentally. She's brain-damaged, isn't she? Sure perhaps she'll become normal . . .'

I thought of shouting at her. Of stopping the car and asking her to get out.

I didn't. I switched off mentally. What else she said I don't remember. But, shrill and grating, the voice went on and on.

Kitchen to sluice room. Trays of snacks. Urinal bottles and bedpans. Calls to the Ward Station; pain situation discussed with nursing staff, with the new influx of medicos who had arrived.

Some were students doing their apprenticeship. Some were graduates on their Internship stint. All were addressed as 'Doctor', and all wore white coats and carried stethoscopes. It was difficult to identify those who had authority to prescribe pain-alleviating drugs.

But I battled on.

The House Surgeon who had exposed my ignorance of Histology was gone. His successor was a harrassed red-headed doctor with an enormous wirey gaucho moustache. He was very earnest and most approachable. He showed concern for his patients as individuals.

An elderly nun occasionally appeared in St Canice's Ward. She went through a ritual of pulling closed Robin's cubicle curtains.

'You know,' she explained, her voice chill, 'the older boys feel embarrassed by this child's nakedness.' Robin's body lay supine on the rubber-covered mattress and foam pad. Often he kicked off the concealing sheet. He found pyjamas a discomfort; they crinkled beneath him in sweat-dried wrinkles.

I made no plea to Robin for modesty. There were enough real problems in his life without making an issue of trivia. When the nun had gone, I pulled open the curtains at his request.

Robin's appetite was increasing. Minced beef sandwiches, barm brack, a little chicken with potatoes.

I suggested turning his bed around so that he could see out onto the lawn and watch the motion of a stripling silver birch which whispered and rustled ceaselessly.

'No. I'll wait until I'm better. It would only remind me of other things. Happy things. I'll wait until I'm home again.' His voice was dreamy. 'Home. Lovely home. No more sickness. No more pain. We'll have to arrange about injections when first I get home . . .'

'We'll do that.' Reassurance.

Once an incredible fourteen hours elapsed with no need for injections. It demolished the theory of drug addiction; that, as had been suggested, he was confusing the craving for morphine with the sensation of real pain.

The red-headed gaucho surgeon tried hard to cope with the changing situations. He prescribed a tranquilliser to alternate with morphine and pethadene. It proved useless.

Occasionally there were good days; comparatively good. Robin extended his reading. Though Bob was still unemployed because of the trade dispute, we managed to keep up the supply of books. Friends helped out by lending. Robin's tastes were changing from fiction. He started to explore a whole range of science and discovery.

Though his physique was deteriorating, his mind and awareness were developing. Our relationship deepened as together we ventured into new worlds outside the confines of the cubicle walls.

'It's lovely to have you here. To make tea and be with me. Won't you stay as long as you can?'

Since sipping from a cup resulted in slopping, I brought in a packet of straws to obviate the drinking problem.

He began to note the progress of other patients. The teenage girl next door on her water mattress: 'She's had chest surgery. Heart, I think it was. I think it's best when you don't know you're going to have an operation. That way you don't have all the fear beforehand.'

His fingers traced the bony ridges of his ribs. 'Soon all these bones will disappear now I'm eating again. I won't be able to see them at all.'

He cocked up his head, supporting it on his hand. 'Look. They cut me there – and there. And again down there. That's three wounds. I think it totals thirty-five stitches altogether.'

He lay back. 'I wouldn't like to be a surgeon. Actually, I think I'm going to be a zoologist. Study animals and birds. Go to Africa. Mum, did you see the little African child up the passage? I've heard the nurses talk about him.'

'Yes. He's coming on nicely. Like you.'

I'd seen him. A small black Botticellian baby with burned leg tissue shrivelled and scarred. His velvet brown eyes watched from his cot.

When times were good, I dreaded the end. Its finality. At least now there was something here. Something breathing, thinking, talking. Some shadow of the Robin he once had been. When he died there would be nothing. A childish voice recorded on a reel of tape; a few photographs. Memories. Nothing more. 'It's so much darker when a light goes out than it would have been if it had never shone.'

Then the pain started again and I desperately wanted the whole ghastly mime to end. There was nothing to break the pain syndrome.

'I'm starving. But every time I eat, I get pain.' The torments of Tantalus. The yearning for food; the exacerbation of the agony.

The writhing body. Teeth biting into dried lips; tiny cracks like bloody fissures. Dehydrated nails, skin creeping up over the cuticles, digging deep into my palms as he counted up to ten at breakneck speed. The syringe emptied. The buttocks were so hard and bony that sometimes the fluid eked out when the needle was withdrawn. A tiny swab of surgical spirit was dabbed vigorously over the puncture. It stung. He winced.

Down the passage, a child sobbed intermittently. 'Mummy, Daddy, I want you.'

'He's been crying all day. His door is closed but still you can hear him a bit,' Robin reported. 'Maybe he had an operation, poor kid.'

'He'll be better in a day or so.'

'I won't have any more operations, sure I won't?' His voice was defensive.

'Why on earth would you? The next thing, you'll be up and getting ready to go home.'

But surgery was on his mind. 'Why did I have so many operations, Mum?'

I thought fast. 'Well, the first was for an appendix. And then there were complications. You had adhesions.' I lied glibly. 'That's when parts of the bowel stick together and cause a blockage and pain. But the last operation cleared them all up. It's only a question of healing now.'

I glanced at the wound. It was ugly. Coarse red blisters were bubbling under the skin.

He looked disturbed. 'I've a strange feeling in my tummy sometimes.'

'It's probably an adhesion on the mend.'

His leg began to twitch uncontrollably. He watched it. 'Sometimes it shivers like that. I don't know why.' The skin lay sagging like webbing over the tendons behind the knobbly upraised knee.

'I don't like this whole business,' he said finally.

At night, the delay in providing injections was aggravated by the staff shortage. My role changed from that of companion to vigilante. I walked the passage obtrusively as the night nurse tried to trace Sr Regina Rosario in an effort to release the drugs.

Robin's agitation grew as our departure time drew nearer.

'Please, please ask her to come quickly if I call. Don't they understand anything? I don't like injections. I don't want them. But the pain gets so terrible. And when there's a delay, it's just agony.'

From his bed he could see the Ward clock suspended over the passage.

'Early this morning, before the day nurses came on, it took twenty-five minutes to get an injection. Sister Rosario was at Mass and the nurse couldn't disturb her in the Chapel, she said. Please won't you try to do something about it?'

Night Nurse was a pleasant shy girl. I spoke to her without much hope of success and reassured Robin before we left.

From the passage, the childish sobbing was louder.

'Mummy, Daddy, I want you . . .' The sound came from a cubicle marked 'Isolation'. A container of special masks was pinned to the door to be used by all who entered his lonely world. A caked putty substance was painted over his neck and chest. In his glass-enclosed island of misery, the sobbing went on . . .

'Mummy, Daddy, I want you. Where are you?'

Robin was despondent.

'Did you hear the news? It's Mr Verkonnen. He's away on holidays. Someone said he's gone to Finland. He'll probably get a cold with the change of climate and won't be back for weeks. How am I ever going to get out of here?'

During the morning, the Surgical Registrar looked in. He was deputising for Mr Verkonnen, in conjunction with Mr Tracey, another Consultant Surgeon.

It was a day of considerable pain. Intense spasms. Repetitive cycles of injections; morphine, pethadene; tranquillisers. Nothing proved effective.

'My tummy's sore. Sore, sore.'

The houseman looked at the wound. It was angry and puffed. The lower stitches were swimming in little puddles of pus.

Mr Tracey came on his Ward Round. He too examined it. The stitches, he felt, should remain in. There was a danger of the wound reopening. He was a cheerful pudgy man with a slight limp. He seemed anxious to help with the problem he had inherited. The charts showed the frequency of injections.

He proffered a new slant on the pain situation. 'Perhaps it's accentuated by your presence. It's possible, you know, that it seems worse to Robin when you are here.'

'Maybe, Mr Tracey, but I don't think so. Occasionally he has fairly long spells without pain.' I took a positive stand. It was not a time for *laissez-faire*. 'Anyway, isn't there any way to eliminate pain completely?

Not just alleviate it? Perhaps give an injection regularly, say every two or three hours?'

'I'll see what I can do,' he promised.

A suppository was inserted. Robin's bowels moved. The bedpan was taken away for examination.

He was restless and fractious.

'I feel awfully queer today. I don't know what it is exactly. Just pretty awful. You can't be as sick as this and ever get better again.'

Pain. It rose in intensity. 'God! Do something quick. It's awful. It's unbearable.' He was screaming fortissimo. 'I want to die right now. Then it will be all over. Do you hear? I want to die. Let me die!'

Sr White came with a syringe. As she removed the needle, the wound bubbled up. It erupted in a flowing rivulet of catarrh-coloured pus. The foul-smelling lava stream gathered momentum as it trickled down Robin's groin on to the sheet.

With professional calm, Sr White assessed the situation and called for nursing help. Supplies were brought from Stores. Thick wads of sterile gamgee; rolls of cotton wool; face masks for the nurses, for myself and Robin.

The smell was nauseating. An overpowering stench of decaying flesh. Robin propped himself on his elbows and watched in mesmeric fascination as the nurses mopped up the flow. *God! What more? To have to watch and smell his own putrefying body!*

Gradually, it drained off. The stitches surfaced again; spikey knots of catgut in pools of pus. The wound was inflamed and tender, but the angry blisters had collapsed.

Robin was alert to everything. He insisted that the stitches must be dried.

Gently Sr White explained. 'Robin, you'll have to be patient. The wound will continue to be moist until all the pus is out. We'll keep it clean for you.'

'It must be healing up inside, mustn't it?' he reasoned stoically.

She nodded.

I choked.

Afterwards, a nurse dressed his upper body in a pyjama top and dried the wet hair. He cooled his forehead and wrists with a cologne stick.

Sr White sprayed the room with air freshener and opened the window. Outside, the staccato chug-chugging of a lawn mower; the scent of cut grass drifted in.

The cubicle was in darkness when I returned that night. Bob was waiting in the Sitting Bay.

'Robin's been asleep for hours. He seems exhausted.'

The gaucho houseman was in the Station. He called me in. 'Robin will feel better now that the wound sepsis is clearing up,' he said. 'That swelling must have been very painful. The inflammation was probably the cause of much of his pain these last few days.'

His humanity touched me. His involvement. *Why, oh why, does it take a newly qualified graduate to see the truth to which others are blind?* Robin's pain was real. Throbbing, torturous and real. It was *not* a condition activated by sympathetic company or craving addiction.

Sr Regina Rosario came into the Ward. She walked to Robin's bed. I followed her. In the eerie glow of the night-light, I realised that if I hadn't known him by the location of his cubicle I would hardly recognise him now as my own child.

She came out. 'The wound is weeping a little.'

I told her of the abscess.

'Yes. And, of course, his healing power is reduced to nil,' she said. 'Although he's eating, he's deriving very little nourishment from it. The sarcoma would be counteracting the effects.'

A compulsion to prise more information made me press on. 'How much longer can he last, Sister?'

'Less than a fortnight, I'd imagine. He'll die of emaciation if it goes on like this.' She tried to salvage some comfort. 'At least, he still has his mind.'

The joy of the intellect. The adventures of the mind. But it couldn't conquer the reality of disease or fear.

Robin lay quietly. Only his wide-awake eyes showed that he wasn't sleeping. As I whispered goodnight, he murmured from the nadir of his suffering.

'What will I do if tomorrow is as bad as today?'

'Tomorrow' came. 6th August 1970.

'Tomorrow' came for Robin. It came with pain.

'Tomorrow', to end all tomorrows came twenty-five years before to a city whose name was little known outside the Orient.

Hiroshima. Hibakuchi – 'the place of suffering'. It came, delivered by a single silver bird, 9,000 lbs birth weight. A ten foot monster, ironically code-named 'little boy'. First-spawned child of Hell on earth under whose mushroom cloud of obscenity Mankind would exist forever more.

'Tomorrow' came for me. Before the mirror I unwound my rollers and saw the coiled strand of tinted hair spring into shape.

A transistorised voice was recalling that day . . .

. . . 'The bomb went off. I threw my daughter flat on the ground. Nothing happened. We thought it must be an explosion. We looked above. We could see this mushroom like a ball of red-smoked fire, whirling like a whirlwind up there. It seemed to extend several miles over the city. Our only immediate after-effects were like a bad suntan. Our noses and ears peeled. Now I suffer from anaemia. The blood cells were affected. I'm on pills every day, with injections fortnightly. That's the way it will always be. But I'm one of the lucky ones . . .'

One of the lucky ones. For, that morning when Hiroshima died, two hundred thousand people ceased to exist.

> 'The bells of hell go ting-aling-aling
> For you but not for me,
> And all the little devils sing-aling-aling . . .'

I chanted the words bitterly, brushing my hair, lacquering it in place with a jet of spray.

'Come on! Let's go off to hospital and watch the torture of children.' My stomach heaved. I felt demented at my own ineptitude to stall the pain syndrome. I was frantic with fear, forboding.

I broke into song again.

> 'Oh death, where is thy sting-aling-aling,
> Oh grave, thy victory?
> The bells of hell go ting-aling-aling . . .'

Bob put a cup of tea on the dressing-table.

I spoke to myself. 'That's right, Inez. Put a brave face on it. Lipstick.

Eyeshadow. Don't let the side down. If you turn on the histrionics, they'll ban you from visiting. So here at home, be your bitchy self. Who the hell can do a thing about it?'

Bob's voice was dead. 'Aren't things bad enough? Do you have to go on like this?'

The tide of tension receded, swept away with the awareness of what I was doing to him. Tears spilled out.

'Bob. What are we going to do?'

'What can we do but go on?'

The phantom of Malcolm's mother passed before my misted eyes. *It's not courage, you know. It's endurance. You just go on because you've no alternative.*

I clung to Bob while he held me. I cried until no tears remained to weep and only convulsive sobs shook my body.

'There. There. Are you better now?'

I nodded. Sipped the cooled tea. Touched silver-blue shadow on my blotched red lids.

'I don't know what I'd do without you, Bob.'

The delays in alleviating Robin's pain were growing longer. He sank deep into apathy. Bony fingers, like human talons, plucked at the identification bracelet. A nurse snipped it with the scissors and threw it into the waste basket. Afterwards I retrieved it – I didn't know why I did it.

Robin watched me. His filmy yellowed eyes focused without interest. An identification bracelet . . .

. . . Blue numerals tattooed indelibly on Semitic skin. No name. Just a number. Shaven heads. First clippers, then a razor. Women's hair for power belts and pipe jointing in U-boats. Sunken eyes in living dead faces. Shuffling gait. Striped pyjama suits. Auschwitz Block 10; experimental surgery on conscious victims, crushed testicles, sterilisation. No names. Just numbers . . .

Nathan gave me tranquillisers. Little white tablets, 2mg Valium. I grew calmer that week.

'You're not doing any good by being here so much, you know,' a doctor said. 'Either to yourself or Robin. It makes it harder for everyone. For Robin, yourselves, the nursing staff.'

I looked into him. He dropped his eyes. 'Perhaps if you just came in for a few minutes each day . . .' His voice faded away limply before my impregnable gaze.

'Yes, doctor. He's your patient. Your medical responsibility. His nuisance value is high. He's taking too long to die. But that cancer-ridden body is not just a name on a chart. It's a child. Our child. He may ultimately die alone. We may not be able to help that. But he will not die feeling he's abandoned.'

'Robin will not die feeling he's abandoned.' I said firmly.

. . . Crucified bodies on barbed wire. Acres of neatly trimmed lawns. White crossed graves in the war cemeteries of France. World War One. World War Two.

. . . Holocausts of Hiroshima. Nagasaki. Crippled lingering deaths from radiation. Counted in millions now.

Yet each man dies alone.

. . . One pilot in a Kamikaze squadron. Final flight to self-destruction on an Allied cruiser.

. . . One Jewish child clutching a bar of soap. Last toddling footsteps through the door of a gas chamber.

Mass extermination.

Yet each makes the final transition alone. Death is the final quintessential Aloneness.

Robin will not die feeling he's abandoned . . .

Robin sucked his thumb, rubbing his upper lip with a tiny square of blanket which he'd used at home as a comforter.

. . . Rhesus monkeys in a laboratory, separated from their mothers. Finding a security substitute in a warm towel.

. . . In the hot sun of the Congo, whole families moved in to the compound of Lambouree hospital. Dr Schweitzer knew the therapeutic value of company. The anguish of mental desolation.

Robin will not die feeling he's abandoned . . .

Pain. Mr Tracey became increasingly embarrassed as I accosted him. He sounded irascible. 'There may be psychological aspects to this pain business.'

I didn't understand but I didn't press him to elaborate. He went on. 'You must leave it to the nursing staff to decide.'

Pain. Twenty minutes of screaming unintelligible sounds. Occasionally a decipherable cry for help. 'Someone do something. Anything. Please kill me.'

Pain. Sr White's off-duty day. The Acting Ward Sister had gone to lunch. Courageous probationers made gallant efforts to trace her in the nurses' canteen, the staff cloakrooms. They drew a blank. She had left the hospital on a shopping trip, it later transpired. The keys to the Dangerous Drugs cupboard of St Canice's were in her pocket.

An elderly nun from another ward came in, carrying a phial, syringe and swabs on a tray.

After the injection, Robin was restless. 'The noise. There's too much noise.'

Blue-grass music, twanged in an Irish-Nashville style, strummed from the Sitting Bay radio. Robin broke into sobs, clapping his hands over his ears. 'Somebody tell them to shut up out there. Keep quiet! Do you hear? Keep quiet!'

Eventually he dozed off. A sleep of subconscious suffering. Each exhalation of breath grated out in a gritty moan that rasped on my raw nerve ends.

Pain. Eight injections between mid-morning and late afternoon. Nausea. He ate nothing for two days; just drank milk diluted with water. Sometimes he vomited.

The nausea troubled him. 'When will this ever end? I feel terribly sick.'

Sr White was concerned. 'We can try to tackle the pain. The vomiting is more difficult.'

He lay sideways; one wasted arm forced his head upright, the other shielded a polythene bowl. His parched lips drooled saliva. Eventually that also dried up. Little grunts. A hiccup of retching. No vomit. For an hour, he forced his weary reflexes to life; dry mouth open, eyes closed, head drooping over the bowl. Occasionally, he jerked upright as sleep tried to capture him.

Afterwards, an aching thirst.

'We'll take the stitches out this afternoon,' Sr White said after Ward Rounds one morning. 'I'll give him a shot of morphine to sedate him before we begin.'

Robin was drowsy as they wheeled in the trolley, but the heavy-lidded eyes opened in instant awareness. Sweaty fingers held mine in a vice clasp.

Sr White bent over his body. Steady hands gripped the wisp of catgut in a forceps. Snip; gently lever, extract. She laid the stitches on a tissue. The wet sutures at the bottom of the wound caused him mental distress but they had been moistened by pus and slipped out more easily than from the scabbed area.

Afterwards he rested and speculated on his recovery. 'I vomited this morning. It comes up in lumps. It's very hard to know what it's safe to eat. I don't seem able to digest anything.'

Bob took over duty. Sr White spoke to me as I was leaving.

'Do you think Robin suspects anything?'

'Definitely he doesn't, Sister.'

'But sometimes he screams that he wants to die . . .'

'Yes. When the pain is very acute,' I interjected. 'But I think it's an interpretation of death as the end of pain at that moment. He feels he'll never be well again. That always he'll be sick and in pain. But he assumes, in between those spasms, that he'll be home sometime. In fact, he's speculated on how he'll manage for injections when he comes home . . .' My voice quavered and began to break. 'He never thinks of death as the end of his life. I'm sure of that.'

As I came in that night, the porter was in loquacious form. He nodded towards Casualty.

'There's an emergency in there, Mrs Heron. Little girl hit by a car. She's bad. Very bad.'

Robin was moaning. Half-asleep. Presently he surfaced.

The Ward was noisy. A parent had brought a crate of Coca Cola for a child's birthday. Bottle tops hurtled along the passage, missiles in a war game.

The pain erupted. An Agency Nurse was on duty in the cubicle next door. A 'special' case. She heard Robin's screams and came in. She telephoned Sr Regina Rosario who was with the casualty case. The Agency Nurse was unafraid, rang repeatedly, unaccustomed to the prolonged delay in palliative procedure.

'This is terrible,' she said, her face lined with concern.

Bob sat with Robin.

I walked the passage.

The Agency Nurse came out of the Station. She had leafed through Robin's charts. 'I can't understand this situation. Surely his drugs could be kept here on the Ward, at night?'

Strengthened by her sympathy, I tramped the warren of passages to Casualty. En route, I met a cortege heading for Theatre. An inert body lay unconscious on a trolley. Nurses rolled a blood transfusion along on a drip-stand.

My quest was hopeless. Cheating death must, in the order of priorities, take precedence over cheating pain.

I returned to St Canice's. Children at play. Child in agony.

Christ! I must do something. Anything. I was suffocating. I opened a window in the Sitting Bay. The Theatre lights were shining.

In his cubicle, Robin was screaming. Writhing. His emaciated body twisted and slithered over the crumpled sheet. His withered arms stretched above his head, gripping the metal bars of the bed.

I felt nausea. Panic.

I turned back to the window. The dusky twilight was misty. Behind me, the agonised body quivered in a macabre dance of torture. Thrashing legs twined, locked like a merman. A yelling cacophony of shrieking humanity.

The nurse was out of sight.

Do it now! I could do it now. Push past Bob. Grab Robin's featherweight in my arms. Dash to the open window. See him wince momentarily as the icy steel frame touched the burning skin. Bundle him through the opening. Release my grip. Split-second drop to oblivion. Red raw meat. Splintered bones. Smashed skull. Pulverised flesh. Splattered blood-drenched body on the shiny wet pavement below.

Christ! What if he didn't die? If, by freak and awful chance, he wasn't killed on impact. If somehow they could scoop up a living breathing composition of molecules and atoms and start a surgical reassembly operation?

. . . Trusting seal-pup on an ice-flow. Clubbed; disemboweled; skinned alive. Gruesome abandoned remains still obscenely living . . .

I closed the window. Turned away.

Forty minutes after the onslaught of pain, the injection came.

. . . The little girl underwent surgery. Before dawn, she died . . .

I pleaded again for help in combating pain. But Mr Tracey's good humour had wilted away. 'You must understand,' he said crisply, 'I've done all I can do.'

Since neither fear nor pain nor drugs had destroyed Robin's mind, we decided to capitalise on his imagination.

We asked permission to bring in goldfish. It was agreed. I bought a plastic tank, clear and shining. It was furnished with multicoloured gravel and wafting ferns. Two fish were netted, flashing gold and silver.

Robin loved it. He instructed me from a handbook on feeding and changing their water.

'I can watch them during the day. And at night, I can hear them,' he said. 'Funny little noises, they make. Nosing in the pebbles for food, I think. I'm sure they can communicate with each other. Ants can, after all. You know, I was looking at them early this morning, shifting through the stones, going in and out through the ferns; and they can fold their top fins down. The fins near the gills keep them moving.'

We played draughts. I noticed he was beginning to outgrow his toys and preferred books and games.

Mr Verkonnen returned and the next day I was called to his consulting rooms. Sr White gave me Robin's file. I took it with me, not daring to detour to the toilets for an illicit perusal.

Mr Verkonnen seemed relaxed. He glanced through the file; then leaned back in his swivel chair.

'Candidly, I was very surprised that Robin is still here. When he was on the operating table he was almost gone. It seemed unlikely he'd last even a week.'

A month had gone by.

Since Mr Verkonnen was being talkative, I bided my time.

He went on to explain that when one operated in a case like Robin's, which was terminal, one used one's discretion as to how much to explore. The massive growth was there, and he had removed part of it. Things were too complicated and extensively affected internally to do more than that.

'Was there a blockage in the intestines?' I braced myself for a truncated reply. But he elaborated further.

The obstruction was not quite complete. A channel was left. A narrow channel which soft foods could get through. But, he added, Robin was eating practically nothing; certainly not enough to sustain life. He would probably grow weaker and, as he had mentioned before, the end would probably be preceded by a slight coma. To a layman, it often seemed like a deep sleep.

'We've played for time, Mr Verkonnen. We told Robin he had adhesions and explained what they are. He seems to accept this.'

He nodded, touching the small square fingers tip to tip. 'That was a good idea.'

'Yes. But if food can't keep him alive indefinitely, how long can he last?'

He glanced at his desk calendar. Quick calculations. Days to death numbered by digits on a diary.

'Mmmm. About three weeks, I would think,' he said finally.

Days drifted by in a doldrum of inactivity. There was no obvious improvement. No regression. In desperation I thought of faith healers. I knew of several from newspaper coverage. But it was an impractical idea and I dismissed it without even mentioning the suggestion to Bob.

One needed faith in faith healers. I lacked it.

I tried to project Robin into a world outside Holy Innocents'. Tried to translocate him from his immediate existence to dreams of a happier future. He responded. Hawaii was our fantasy that became a mythical reality.

A friend had settled on Oahu Island. He was a retired airline pilot and he knew of Robin's illness. A stream of postcards, leaflets, travel brochures and pamphlets came by airmail.

Aloha! Pineapples, salt-water geysers, blanched coral atolls. Erupting volcanoes and black-sand beaches.

A century of benign monarchy. Six thousand square miles of bewitching beauty. Diamond Head. We talked of times we would spend at the pilot's home and studied photographs of a bungalow, palm-sheltered, wave-caressed, at the ocean's edge. Recuperative sun-drenched days. Warm purple nights.

Kama-Hoa-Lii. Legendary shark king, re-incarnation of a Hawaiian fisherman. Great God of the Sea. Pearl Harbor; archaeological evidence of a marine amphitheatre where Olympian games were held in his honour. Zeus of the Pacific. His palace a subaqueous cave in the blue waters of Honolulu. He watched over fishermen in danger and guided them back to safe anchorage.

Kama-Hoa-Lii. Kaanapali. Waikiki. The melody of word sounds in music. Dream sounds.

At night, when Robin was sleeping, I wrote brief notes and left them by his pillow.

'. . . sleep well, Robin. See you in Hawaii.'

Life lived vicariously. "Dreams are true while they last, and do we not live in dreams?"

'Hold my hand. Just hold my hand.' After the pain abated, Robin lay quietly, his damp fingers in mine. 'I want you to be with me always. When you die, you'll wait for me and then we'll be happy together in heaven.'

His simple sincerity stripped the words of sentimentality. I gulped back the familiar burning knot of sadness, savouring the relief of his assumption that I would be the first to die.

The Chaplain visited the Ward each day. Bob was concerned that perhaps Robin should be receiving Holy Communion. He mentioned it to the priest who broached the subject with Robin. The response was unenthusiastic. Robin told Bob about it.

'There's the business of fasting. And sometimes I'm asleep in the morning. They'd only wake me up and then there might be pain. And there's all that trouble of a little Mass at the bottom of the bed.'

Bob relayed this to the Chaplain.

'It's not a Mass, of course. The ciborium and pyx are brought around. That's all.' He continued, 'However, I don't know about the medical aspects. The fasting could be dispensed with but I'm not sure if Robin would be able to receive the Host.'

I remembered Religious Knowledge classes. A nun's earnest voice. Reverent. 'If someone vomits up the Communion wafer, the priest must gather up the fragments of the Sacred Body and consume them himself.' I had experienced a guilty sense of revulsion . . .

Sr White had doubts. She suggested that if Robin mentioned Holy Communion, it could be considered.

He didn't refer to it again.

Sr Regina Rosario finished her stint of Night Duty. Sr Dolorosa took over. I had hoped for an improvement in the nocturnal pain situation.

Hope died that first night.

'Things are no better,' Robin said next morning. 'Sister Dolorosa was making out reports and couldn't be disturbed. It was ages before she came.'

'Don't worry. We'll tackle it.'

'Nuns seem more casual than nurses, I think,' he commented.

'Well, their hours are long. They've a lot of responsibility, particularly at night; and when they're very busy, they get impatient like anyone else.'

'But aren't they something special?'

'Yes. It's not just a job. They don't get paid for it. They give their lives to helping others.'

'Well, I don't think Sister Regina Rosario or Sister Dolorosa deserve to be nuns at all,' Robin said decisively.

'They mean well,' I replied, trying not to let my prejudices colour my judgment.

I lay in bed, listening to the wind rattling the windows. It had risen to gale force.

After an outburst of depressive weeping, Bob tried to reason with me. 'What exactly is it you find so hard to accept? Robin's death or the suffering?'

I struggled to verbalise unexpressible feelings. 'It's the waste of his life. Not his value to others; but the loss of his potential to himself. Last week, a girl threw herself off a bridge over the M.1. She was killed. She was about sixteen; a drug addict, and there was no clue to her identity. Officially, a nobody from nowhere. Obviously she had gargantuan psychological problems with which she could no longer cope. She made her decision, however desperate. But at least she'd had her chance of life. To live it or destroy it, for herself.'

Bob was silent.

'Don't you see what I mean?' I continued. 'Robin will never have his chance.'

'It would be so much easier for you if you had faith in God's Will.'

'Does it trouble you that I can't believe?'

His voice was sad. 'It disappoints me, I suppose.'

'At least I've tried. I've read over the years. I read as much as I've time to, as much as my brain will absorb at the moment.'

'I know. But why don't you read Catholic philosophers?' he asked reasonably.

'Because, by very definition, Christians are partisan. They are writing and thinking subjectively. I've tried C. S. Lewis. He was an agnostic who described himself as 'the most reluctant convert in England'. But I found his *Problem of Pain* unconvincing and inconclusive. Bertrand Russell, on the other hand, was a Christian who couldn't reconcile faith with logic or reason. He wandered into rejection and proceeded from that to find a way to what, for him, was truth.'

Bob paused. 'Life is so much harder for you, isn't it? You think so much. You feel so much.'

'People reckon that you feel it all just as deeply. It's just that you say less.'

He shook his head. 'No. You've more awareness, I think. More sensitivity. Emotions are intensified for you. You experience greater happiness than I do and greater depths of misery. I move on a more even keel.'

'Maybe we complement each other.'

It was a good marriage. Quiet. Contented. Companionable. Too weary now for passion.

Suffering, it is reckoned, can be measured in several dimensions. Mental, physical, psychological and economic. We were now experiencing it in all four forms.

The mental and physical pain affected everyone. The psychological was less overt. Despite the financial strain of Bob's unemployment, we paid the hospital account weekly – drawing on reserves which we had saved as long-term security for Helen's uncertain future. Bob's annual salary, when he was working, was in excess of the figure which entitled Robin to free medical care. So, by definition, he was a 'private patient'.

The hospital account covered maintenance. Nothing more. Drugs, Theatre and surgical fees all would be presented when Robin's file was closed. Maintenance meant food and nursing. But at least by paying for it promptly, Robin was entitled to receive it.

Money couldn't buy back his health. But it could provide him with some degree of comfort and consideration.

The Jelly Incident proved that. And it was catalytic.

Jelly. Boiling water poured over a synthetically coloured, artificially flavoured tablet of gelatine. A few pence. An inexpensive convenience food. Yet it triggered off a problem.

Sometimes there would be a plate of jelly left over in the Ward kitchen. More often than not, some youngster would feel peckish between tea-time and breakfast next morning. The jelly would vanish. Robin developed a craving for it.

One evening, with the Night Nurse's permission, I made a sortie to the hospital kitchens on the ground floor. They were a great acreage of pantries, sculleries, ante-rooms – all scrupulously clean and shining, and gleaming with huge machines for vegetable peeling, cooking, washing up.

It was in darkness. Armed with a bowl and spoon from St Canice's, I blundered past stoves and worktops. I found my way to the row of refrigerators and tried the heavy doors. The first was locked. Like a ravenous Goldilocks, I tried the next. A padlock dangled from the handle. I pulled the door and it opened. An automatic light illuminated the interior.

It was a walk-in refrigerator. Great quasi-cattle troughs of jelly lined the shelves. Triumphantly, I scooped the surface and loaded up a bowl of wobbling booty.

Robin attacked it with relish. As it slithered down his throat, the Night Nurse came in and sat on his bed.

'Was anyone on duty in the kitchens?' she asked.

'Not a soul about. I just pottered around and helped myself.'

'Just as well,' she remarked. 'There's not much love lost between the catering staff and the nurses at the moment. Relationships are a bit strained.'

She took up Robin's empty dish. 'It's easier all round if you can get Robin's jelly for yourself,' she said.

The jelly routine became a nightly ritual. An uneventful expedition until the night I surprised one of the kitchen staff. She was sitting in a dimly-lit scullery, a pot of tea steaming on the table. It must have been an illicit venture on her part as well, for her instinctive reaction was to sally out from the shadows and attack. I was heading unobtrusively for the fridge when she forayed forth. A clumping middle-aged woman in check carpet slippers.

'What are you doing here?' Suspicion reeked from her voice and face.

I stood guiltily, holding the empty plate and spoon. Then I started a spate of explanations.

'It's my son, you see. He's a patient in St Canice's Ward. He wanted jelly and there was none up there. It seemed to be all right for me to collect it from here.' I tried to sound nonchalant.

'I can't allow it.'

Anger rose like a bubble. I tightened my grip on the spoon. *Keep cool!*

'Then let's pretend you didn't see me. You know nothing about it. I don't exist. Or, if there's any trouble, you can say I insisted. I'll take the responsibility. Okay?' I moved forward.

She blocked my path. Her voice rose truculently. 'The fridges are locked at night. I have the key.'

'That's all right. I'll manage.'

'I said they're locked.'

'And I said I'll manage.' The spoon became a weapon in my hand. I could have eviscerated her with pleasure as she stood there. A maverick queen of the kitchens; a solid bulwark of authority between the empty plate and the jelly troughs.

'One of the fridges is open and I'm going to help myself. That's it.'

White-hot fury ripped through me like a laser beam. We had paid for food and nursing care to the tune of several hundred pounds. I would be damned if anyone or anything would stand between a dying child and a few pence worth of jelly.

Confrontation; capitulation.

She sensed the incipient violence emanating from me. Without a word, she slouched off into the darkness.

Robin had his jelly.

Dreams of Hawaii couldn't banish the reality of pain when it struck at 3.00 a.m.

Robin was trembling with distress as he told me of it next morning.

'Sister Dolorosa came in shortly after you had left. She was very nice. Chatted about the goldfish and looked at my books. But when I got pain, she was making out her reports, the nurse said. It was forty minutes before she came with an injection. Mum, is there nothing you can do about it? Please, please, do something. You've just got to do something.'

There was something. Monitoring Robin's suffering and alleviating it when possible had become my *raison d'etre*. I could storm the Bastille. Rock the established *status quo*.

I took out a pen and drafted a letter to Matron.

'Matron wants to see you,' a young nurse whispered in my ear. Robin was sleeping. I was dozing in an easy chair which I'd brought from the Sitting Bay into his cubicle.

'She wants to see you. Matron does.' the nurse murmured again more urgently. A few days had elapsed since I'd left my letter at the switchboard.

The nurse piloted me to Matron's office and knocked gently on the door. Then she ushered me in. Matron was taking a phone call. She interrupted it to politely acknowledge introductions. I braced myself and waited.

My letter lay on the desk. Familiar typescript, as succinct and comprehensive as I could make it. Two paragraphs of introduction to Robin's history at Holy Innocents'. With several hundred patients in her charge, she could not be expected to keep a mental dossier on each case.

In my final paragraphs, I'd expressed appreciation of the efficiency of her nursing staff, mentioning several by name – girls whose exceptional kindness and dedication merited special commendation.

The guts of the letter lay on the middle page.

I had traced the pain syndrome, the time lag of injections at night. I had confined my statements to those occasions when I had personally been there, in late evening, and witnessed the delays.

I knew that, under the Dangerous Drugs' Act, strict regulations pertained to the custody of such drugs as morphine and pethadene. My plea was that perhaps some arrangement could be made whereby the relevant drugs could be left conveniently available to be administered, when necessary, as expeditiously as possible.

It had not been an easy letter to write. But I felt it would be a violation of my own probity and my duty to Robin if I didn't do something tangible to try to rectify the situation which was resulting in such prolonged periods of pain.

'. . . Robin's life is waning,' I had written, 'and my only hope is that what time is left to him may be as peaceful as possible. The only thing which we now can give him is our company, our time, and our endeavours to alleviate his suffering . . .'

Matron was a tall woman with narrow patrician features and an aquiline nose. Her whitening hair was partially concealed under the veil of a nursing nun. But her face was a contradiction of her manner; she radiated friendliness and concern.

'Sit down, Mrs Heron,' she invited, replacing the receiver. 'I'm sorry about delaying you.'

I took the proffered chair.

'I know the trauma it has been for you these past months,' she said, glancing at the typewritten pages. 'Your letter is very explanatory. Now, as to the drugs situation.'

The problem, she felt, might have been due to the change-over of Night Sisters. Sometimes it took a little while to sort these things out.

I listened. But I was unconvinced.

Finally, I interjected. 'Perhaps so, Matron. But it's a pattern that's been evolving for quite some while. And the time lag doesn't occur only at night, I'm afraid.'

She was sympathetic, in her silence.

Then she asked gently. 'Has your son any idea that he's dying?'

'None at all. We always talk positively of the future. Of the time when he'll be back home and things will be normal again.'

'Maybe he does know,' she suggested softly. 'Often children sense death is coming. But they have no fear. Only sympathy for their parents.'

Tears welled in my eyes. I forced them back. Robin's cause could not be jeopardised by having me branded as a pain-phobist.

She stood up. 'Well, thank you for writing to me. I'll certainly see what can be done.'

There it ended. Hers was the final repository of power.

I filled Sr White in on the details of my talk with Matron.

'We've been wondering, some of the nurses and myself, if you ever thought of taking Robin home,' she said.

The suggestion surprised me. 'That's off-the-record, I'm guessing?'

She smiled agreement. 'It was just our own speculation. I mean, it must be costing the earth to keep him here. You're even bringing in some of your own food supplies to him. And there's nothing we're doing that couldn't be done by nurses in your own home.'

'Actually, we have talked of it – Bob and I,' I admitted. 'But we dismissed the idea for two reasons. We'd need three shifts of nurses to cover the twenty-four hours; that would work out more expensive than here. And secondly, while we're accustomed to Robin's physical appearance, it could be terrifying for our other children. His brother Billie is seven. He's the one most likely to be affected. Helen is brain-damaged, so it's unlikely she'd notice. And Michael is only a baby. But Billie's shock at Robin's changed appearance could register in his face and give Robin a clue to what lies ahead for him.' I hesitated, then said spontaneously, 'But thank you for taking me into your confidence.'

Next day Mr Verkonnen came on his Ward Rounds. He said nothing to me but moved out on to the passage for a confabulation. The gaucho-moustached house surgeon, Mr Tracey and Sr White surrounded him, heads nodding in a silent mime. It lasted quite a while. Eventually they left.

As I passed the Ward Station en route home, Sr White called me in. Time and respect had bonded a mutual trust.

'Today, Mr Verkonnen asked me what I thought,' she began, her fingers adjusting the dark knot of hair under her lace cap. 'I said that, to me, Robin seems weaker sometimes. Then he rallies.'

'And what did Mr Verkonnen think?' I prompted.

'Well, he asked details of vomiting, bowel motions, diet, etcetera.

But he passed no comment.' She continued: 'He doesn't like the quantities of morphine and pethadene. Largactil has been suggested. It can be given orally or by injection. You know, I've a feeling it could be with a view to sending Robin home.'

Bob and I mulled it over afterwards.

From the trickle of information that was leaking out to us, it seemed that medical opinion was as flummoxed as we were ourselves.

That night I telephoned Nathan. He listened. Then questioned me. 'It's certainly strange,' he said finally. 'Children usually go very quickly after surgery which reveals hopeless malignancy.'

Robin had held on to life for an incredible ten weeks since his first operation.

His grip still seemed a long way from slipping.

A goodwill had been established with the Night Porter. We came and went without question. Sometimes he stood at the hospital entrance door and chatted ruminatively.

One night, as we were leaving, Mr Verkonnen passed us in the hall. He made no sign of recognition but hurried on towards the Theatres. The porter was in voluble mood. 'I see Mr Verkonnen has been called in. Must be emergency surgery,' he reflected.

I nodded agreement, one hand on the door. He came out and joined us on the steps.

He went on. 'Well do I remember when he was a student and him coming in here on his bike, with his briefcase slung over the handlebars.'

It was an incongruous picture when equated with the tailored suits and immaculate white cuffs of the Consultant Surgeon we knew.

'He's a very good surgeon,' he continued, 'even if he is a bit short on the small talk.'

Next day I made an appointment to see Mr Verkonnen.

The chair to which he gestured had no arm rests. It could have placed one at a psychological disadvantage; fiddle with one's fingers? sit on one's hands? I did neither, for this time I had come equipped with a notebook and a list of salient questions.

I explained my idiosyncrasy as one of a journalist's occupational hazards, an obsession with detail which might otherwise be forgotten.

He smiled and waited.

I began. 'Robin vomits only occasionally. He has bowel motions about twice weekly . . .' I became conscious that it sounded like a clinical inventory, but I went on. 'Would this indicate an arrest of the growth. I mean, *you* know what the third operation revealed. Was the growth confined, or had it spread, or is it likely to spread?'

He leaned forward slightly and explained that what he had found, and could still feel physically with his hand, was a very big growth on the back abdominal wall.

'Is further surgery ruled out?' I half-dreaded the possible reply.

'It's highly unlikely.'

'Robin's having a lot of pain, Mr Verkonnen. Is he likely to become more distressed and experience more discomfort before the end?'

The pain, Mr Verkonnen felt, might not be as severe as one might think. The intestines were now very limp. Instead of pulsating and pushing the matter along as they normally would, things were just slipping through. There wouldn't be any pressure from a pushing motion. So the pain should not be so terribly severe.

'It's real to Robin,' I said.

He agreed. But the worst of it was over now, he reckoned. At the beginning, there had been the wound itself. Then came the abscess when, naturally, the pain was very acute.

I said nothing; remembering the days before the abscess broke when the pain was thought to be partially psychological. That was now history.

I looked at my notebook.

Mr Verkonnen paused, as though considering how much more to volunteer. Then he went on to speak of the drugs. Robin, it seemed, had been getting morphine and pethadene with increasing frequency. There could be a danger, particularly with morphine, that he might have hallucinations. 'They could be extremely disturbing,' he added.

The blue eyes below the white-blond hair were watching me. I changed direction.

'Once again, Mr Verkonnen, how much longer will Robin have to endure all this?'

He folded his hands tidily. Not more than a few weeks, he estimated.

Muscular deterioration would eventually bring things to a standstill. The muscles just wouldn't be able to absorb any more. It wouldn't actually be the heart that would give up, but a sort of starvation.

'Yes, but Robin is eating,' I reminded him. Then I listed the hospital fare, augmented by yoghurt, biscuits and orange juice with which we supplemented his diet.

Mr Verkonnen nodded. The muscles would not be transmuting the food into substance that was any good to Robin. He judged the calorie intake to be about 800 per day. It should be about 2500. But he made a note to have a check made on it.

I glanced at the last question in my notebook. Then I chose my words with care.

'If surgery is unlikely,' I said, 'what about radium or other treatment?'

Mr Verkonnen answered that he had considered it and ruled it out. He politely guided me to the door.

It was over a year before I met him again. Robin's case was closed by then.

Sr White saw me viewing the bottle of syrup which stood on Robin's locker.

'It's pretty powerful,' she said. 'I worked once with alcoholics. It was used for heavy sedation. They'd be woken for meals, then off to sleep again.'

Robin showed the effects. He lay, eyes half-closed. His breathing was noisy, hissing out. But the pain still penetrated the drug-induced sleep. His voice rose in crescendos of agony.

'Oh God! Will someone ever come? It's terrible. It's waves and waves of pain and I can't keep quiet. Someone do something. Quick!'

Five injections between mid-morning and early afternoon. His wasted buttocks bled after each puncture.

In the evening, his bowels moved without the aid of suppositories.

The dietitian called. A slender girl with swinging fair hair and an aloof manner.

'Sr White tells me you've been bringing in food for this patient.' She nodded towards Robin's cubicle. My actions sounded criminally suspect. I refused to be drawn into polemics. She went on. 'I want to check his calorie intake. You will have to keep a check on his exact diet over twenty-four hours, starting today. You'll need to keep a list of precisely what you supply to him.'

I agreed. Bananas, jelly, chicken and vegetables; Ryvita, Snack biscuits, yoghurt and orange juice. The miscellany of cartons and wrappings grew with the passing hours. After lunch the next day, a nurse collected them for assessment. It was Saturday. A September Saturday. It was unlikely that we would know her findings before Monday.

Sunday was a litany of suffering. Ampule after ampule was emptied into the tortured upper quadrant of his buttocks. Finally, the wasted flesh rejected the palliative fluid. Blood and serum trickled out. A nurse injected the needle into the sagging skin of Robin's leg. He writhed and screamed in agony.

'Oh Christ! Not my leg. Oh no! No!'

Sweat ran down the deeply sculptured lines of suffering that scarred his haggard face. His hair was saturated. His eyes were flaming red sockets of scalding tears.

The pattern of delays continued through the evening. The Night Nurse manfully tried to cope. There was an emergency in Cherubims' Ward. She phoned for help. I accosted a distracted House Surgeon as he pushed open the swing doors into the infants' area.

'We're understaffed,' he said tersely. 'There's nothing I can do at the moment.' The doors swung closed behind him.

In St Canice's, Robin's screams were ear-piercing, shattering the other children's sleep. Some became restless, tossing listlessly in their beds.

Robin lost control of his bladder and urinated in the bed. There was a shortage of sheets in the linen cupboard. The nurse brought a folded pile of draw-covers as an impromptu substitute. It was impossible to attempt to remove the soaked sheet. Robin twisted and contorted. Bony knuckles shone silver-white through the translucent skin as his fists hammered on the bed. Toes gripped the wet cotton. His torso arched upwards, revealing sores on his buttocks and the raw spinal vertebrae.

All the time he shrieked. Brain pounded by pain. Agonised animal yells as the body protested.

After fifty minutes, Night Sister came with an injection.

It was too late. I had crossed the Rubicon.

Robin slept. The nurse made a pot of tea. I waited immobile in the Sitting Bay. As calmly and objectively as possible, I tried to view the situation. At Holy Innocents', things had reached an impasse. But there were other hospitals. Other doctors. There must be something more we could do.

At home that night, I telephoned Nathan.

Nathan initiated us in medical protocol. We learned the procedures involved in calling in another opinion to see Robin. He named the consultants at several cancer hospitals.

'A Consultant Radiotherapist, that's what you're looking for. Dr Monaghan is a very good man. He's at Bramble Grange.'

We made our decision. The days of complacency were over.

Any fears of my own cowardice were dispelled when I arrived at St Canice's Ward next morning.

Sr White broke the news to me. 'Mr Verkonnen has gone away on holidays,' she began. 'None of us knew anything about it. Usually he tells us that Mr Tracey will be looking after his patients. But this time, he didn't say anything to us.'

'Did he leave any instructions about Robin?' I asked.

'Only to let things go on as they're going, his houseman said.'

It was too nebulous for my taste. 'And the dietitian's report, Sister?'

'Yes! It came through this morning,' she answered. 'Robin's calorie intake was 2100.'

That made a total of 1300 in excess of Mr Verkonnen's impromptu assessment. I told Sr White of our plans.

Next morning, I moved into action. From home, I telephoned the Holy Innocents' Consultants' Clinic – pre-planned strategy to start at the top of the structure.

'I'd like to make an appointment with Mr Verkonnen, please. It's in connection with his patient, Robin Heron.' I knew the answer; but the formalities had to be observed.

'He's away at the moment,' his secretary explained.

'Well, perhaps I could see Mr Tracey?'

'He won't be in here for a couple of days. Not until Thursday. You could contact him at his private rooms, but he won't have the files there.'

'It's rather urgent, I'm afraid,' I persisted.

'Then you'd best get in touch with the Surgical Registrar,' she answered.

'And how do I do that, please?'

'I can't transfer the call. But if you telephone the hospital again, they'll put you through.'

I dialled Holy Innocents' a second time and was linked up with Out-Patients Department.

I asked to speak with the Surgical Registrar. The secretary was un-certain. 'I'm not sure if he's here right now. Hold on and I'll see.' She covered the mouthpiece; muffled sounds of conversation.

Her voice came back on the line. 'He's extremely busy,' she said pithily.

'Right.' It was not a time for procrastination. 'Would you please explain to him that I am Robin Heron's mother. That we would like to call in another opinion on Robin's case. As we understand it, the consultant of our choice must be invited by some member of the staff at Holy Innocents'. Mr Verkonnen is away. Perhaps the Surgical Registrar would contact me, either at St Canice's Ward or at home, as soon as is convenient for him. I'll give you the phone number. It's urgent and important.'

More blanketed sounds behind the mouthpiece. Then she spoke with finality. 'He will be busy all day in Theatre. I suggest you phone St Canice's Ward.'

My call to St Canice's was put through. I asked for the House Surgeon on duty. He was in Casualty but he phoned back within minutes. I recognised his voice; the red-haired gaucho-moustached doctor.

I explained our request and the problem I was having in contacting any of the Holy Innocents' consultants. I continued. 'I know medical protocol. That, according to etiquette, a member of the staff must invite in another opinion.' I paused for the next thrust, 'But I also know that a hospital cannot refuse such a request. I've looked into this – and we know where we stand. I don't mean that to sound unpleasant; just firm.'

There was a brief silence. I continued, 'Perhaps *you* would be able to call in a second opinion, doctor?'

He seemed amused, as though enjoying the power politics being played safely above his head. 'I'm afraid, Mrs Heron, I'm far too low down the line to do that,' he demurred.

'And I'm sure your modesty is quite unjustified and doesn't reflect your abilities,' I parried.

He said, with a smile in his voice, 'Look, I'll explain to the Surgical Registrar and get him to contact you.'

Reverberations echoed along the grapevine.

Within a few hours, Mr Tracey, who wasn't scheduled to be in Holy Innocents' for two days, knocked at the cubicle door.

I explained the position.

'I consider it a reasonable request,' the surgeon said, his face showing interest. Then, more cautiously, 'Does Mr Verkonnen know of your intentions?'

I kept my tone neutral. 'We have had no contact with Mr Verkonnen since I saw him before the calorie intake check was done last week.'

'I see.' His voice was equally non-commital.

Sr White was monitoring developments with interest. She explained that radium treatment had been discussed; that Mr Tracey felt it could give a remission, but as he wasn't Robin's surgeon, he couldn't make the decision. 'However,' she cautioned, 'there is one thing. Be sure to establish that Robin can return here afterwards, if necessary. It might be awkward for you, as Mr Verkonnen's away and hasn't okayed the transfer – if it materialises.'

With sincerity I thanked her. We owed her much. But if Robin was to leave Holy Innocents' alive, I promised myself that he would not return there.

That afternoon, Mr Tracey dropped in again. Bob was sitting with Robin.

'I've contacted Dr Monaghan of Bramble Grange Hospital,' Mr Tracey said. 'He'll come and see Robin tomorrow.'

Dr Monaghan didn't wait until next day.

That evening, he came to Holy Innocents'.

FOUR

September, October

'See the wretch that long has tost
   On the thorny bed of pain,
At length repair his vigour lost
   And breathe and walk again:
The meanest floweret of the vale,
The simplest note that swells the gale,
The common sun, the air, the skies,
To him are opening Paradise.'
Thomas Gray (*Ode on the Pleasure arising from Vicissitude*)

Dr Monaghan was devoid of pretentions. He was sartorially undistinguished, with a thin vulpine face and a gentle unassuming manner.

He knocked at Robin's cubicle door and checked my relationship to his new patient. As a prelude, he chatted to Robin, commenting on the goldfish, asking him of his interests and hobbies. Then he rubbed his hands together, stimulating the circulation.

'I don't want to chill your skin with my cold touch,' he explained. A physical examination started. With extraordinary gentleness, his fingers ran over the naked emaciated body; lingered on the neck and under-arms where the lymph glands are located.

'How long ago is it since he was X-rayed?' he asked.

'About seven weeks, I think.' I had learned never to make an arbitary statement. 'Before the third operation. None since then, as far as I know.'

'I'll arrange for another,' he said decisively.

In the Ward Station, I saw him scrutinising Robin's file. Head down, he turned the pages. Reading; pausing. Some time later he looked up and beckoned me out to the passage.

'We'll have him transferred to Bramble Grange tomorrow. I'm going to start him on Ray Treatment.'

I asked no details. Sufficient that things were moving fast.

His voice was kind. 'I cannot promise you a cure,' he warned, 'but I am certain we can do a great deal to help him.'

He went in to speak to Robin. 'Would you be willing to come to my hospital, Robin?' he asked. 'We specialise in curing pain.'

Robin's wrinkled face broke into smiles.

That night, I took the suitcase of funeral clothes home and unpacked them.

Bramble Grange was a five-minute drive from our home. We feared that Robin might associate its name with cancer so we falsified the truth a little.

'Many diseases are treated there. Things like your adhesions, for example. They use a "lamp" treatment. It's completely painless and very effective.'

'Good,' Robin sounded cheerful, 'and Dr Monaghan will be looking after me, won't he? I like him. He's very friendly and he doesn't fuss.'

We settled the final account for maintenance at Holy Innocents' and Sr White made the necessary travel arrangements.

'An ambulance will call early in the afternoon,' she said. 'Bramble Grange have phoned us and confirmed that a single room is available for Robin.'

This would be slightly more expensive than a general ward but it had the advantage of privacy. Robin was accustomed now to being alone. When bouts of pain struck, it would be less distressing for him and for the other patients.

I put the goldfish tank and his books into the car and drove to Bramble Grange. It was beautifully located in the foothills of the mountains. An old mansion in wooded parklands.

Aesthetically, it was architectural perfection. The original house formed the nexus of the hospital complex which opened out in bright airy wings from the central building. A stream wandered through the grounds and flowed into a lake. The gardens were panoramically landscaped; a harmony of stone and trees and dark water. They were ablaze with September colours.

A uniformed attendant directed me into the car park, shaded under a colonnade of splendid copper beeches.

Robin's room was on the top floor of a two-storey wing. 'No 12. Ward P', midway down a corridor which opened from the Nurses' Station. The window offered a view of the Admission area and the flower-lined path to the car park. Outside, patients in dressing-gowns were enjoying the sunshine. A small child sat in a wheelchair, shaded by an almond tree.

I scattered Robin's treasures around the room, personalising it for his arrival. It looked cosy with none of the clinical chill of a hospital. The walls were papered in soft pink. A multi-channel television set stood on a fitted cupboard. There were rugs and easy chairs, and light brackets over the washbasin and the bed. I found a shadowed shelf to accommodate the goldfish out of direct daylight.

'I'm sure you'd like a cup of tea while you're waiting,' a nurse said, carrying in a tray.

She tucked two hot water bottles into the bed. A sponge mattress had been provided.

Before diesel power usurped their cabled transport, the ambulance men had been tram drivers. On the journey to Bramble Grange, they regaled Robin with stories of the past. My mother travelled with him.

Robin was breathless with excitement as his stretcher was wheeled in. 'Sr White came down to see me off from Holy Innocents'. The curtains were drawn in the ambulance, but Grannie would say, "Guess where we are now?" and it was great. I loved feeling the throbbing of the engine again and everything.'

He was cocooned in blankets, a tiny geriatric Rip Van Winkle, a weird wizened gnome-child. His wan face peered out, head slowly swaying like a very old tortoise.

He was lifted on to the bed. Pyjama-clad, he lay back on the smooth white sheets. He was exhausted but his eyes travelled round the room, radiating happiness. A nurse appeared with a menu. There was a choice of five items for tea. He was hungry but apprehensive that a pain problem would start if he ate.

Dr Monaghan came in. He had the curious shuffling walk of those who like to be inconspicuous. His words dispelled Robin's fears.

'Now don't worry. We'll cope with that. You know, old man, you've had an awful lot of those blooming drugs. We'll have to do something about it. We're going to give you tablets if you have pain.'

The drugs, he explained, were kept in the D.D. cupboard in the Nurses' Station just a few yards away. If the tablets were ineffective, injections could be administered promptly.

'I'm not going to do anything at all with you this evening, Robin. You've had quite sufficient activity for one day. But tomorrow we'll start the treatment.'

The bedrest was pulled out and a trolley with Robin's tea tray was rolled up in front of him. He poured from the teapot and drank from the cup. Then, he set to work with a knife and fork. 'Look! It's real china. Not polythene things.'

Mesmerised, I watched. For over seven weeks he had been lying supine, sipping liquids through a straw. This change was incredible; but true.

Later the pain started. The tablets proved ineffective. Quickly a palliative injection was provided.

Robin spent the evening watching television. At suppertime, the Night Nurse brought milk and biscuits. Just before 10.00 pm, she came with a trolley of equipment. His dressings were changed. The variegated bruises on his flanks were soothed with an emollient and cream was applied to the red blotched ankles and elbows. The sheets were smoothed and his pillows plumped up, the blankets straightened. A night-light, at floor level, was switched on. The electric bell was placed beside his head, within easy reach.

Robin snuggled down contentedly.

Twice during the night he had pain. It was treated promptly with tablets. The pain passed.

In addition to the specialised personnel, Bramble Grange had a visiting staff which included a gynaecologist, a physician, a dental surgeon and a laryngologist. There was also a panel of several eminent surgeons drawn from the leading city hospitals.

The clinics covered the country. Suspect patients were referred by local doctors to the visiting consultant radiotherapists and were, when necessary, transferred to Bramble Grange.

There, in the Diagnositic X-ray Department, their cases were studied. Two main Theatres were available for surgery. The Deep X-ray Therapy Department provided radium and cobalt treatment. There were several Pathology Laboratories and a Physics staff were engaged in the planning, maintenance and checking of radio-active isotopes and other lethal substances.

It was a small hospital; one hundred and fifty beds. The turnover was fairly quick. In the old mansion, there was a hostel for ambulatory patients domiciled outside the city. Once their treatment was completed for the day, they were free to go out to visit friends, go shopping in town, or wander down to the local pubs for a congenial drink.

It was generously staffed. Ward P carried a ratio of fifteen nurses to twenty patients. Allowing for off-duty and holiday periods, it meant that only rarely were they working under pressure. Ward orderlies helped with bedmaking, serving meals and routine patient care. All the nurses were qualified and equal in rank so none of the fear of trainees for seniors existed. On Staff Sister's day off, one of the others deputised for her.

The emphasis was on the patients' mental and physical welfare. The active walked down to the Deep X-ray Therapy Department for treatment. The less mobile were pushed in wheelchairs. The severely ill were wheeled along in their beds.

Relief of pain was the first priority, to rehabilitate patients for a return to as full and normal a life as possible.

All this I learned from observation and from a leaflet given to me by the hospital almoner.

The night of Robin's transfer to Bramble Grange, I dropped in on Nathan. It was very late. He waved my apologies aside.

A warm glow of firelight flickered in the grate. I sat, relaxed, on the hearth rug.

'Can I ask you a few questions?'

He smiled indulgently. 'Go ahead. I'll try and answer. Are we going to delve into metaphysics, the numinosum, or medicine?'

'Medicine tonight, please. God has ceased to exist for me. Either he's a myth created by man's necessity, or he's a monster unworthy of acknowledgment let alone adoration . . .' I glanced up. 'I'm not hurting you by airing these views, am I, Nathan?'

The warmth of affection shone in his ageing eyes. 'You couldn't hurt me, Inez, because you would never deliberately intend to. But we'll agree to disagree about God. You know, you may be much nearer to Him than you recognise yourself to be. Yours is the hard road and I speak from experience. But now I am at peace.'

He leaned back from the firelight. The worn springs of his chair squeaked. 'So it's to be medicine. Where do we begin?'

'Tell me something about cancer!'

'That's a tall order. However, let's relate it to Robin's case for a start.'

'Right! Then we begin with a lymphosarcoma.' I waited. But there was no tension in any subject, or in silence, when shared with this man.

He stood up and moved along the bookshelves. His back was to me as he searched. 'Cancers take many many forms, you know. In themselves, even in different parts of the world.' He fumbled a moment. 'Ah yes! here we are.' He handed me a medical dictionary. 'Take that home with you. It'll explain quite a lot, when you've time to browse through it.'

I thanked him.

'Dr Monaghan speaks of treatment. Is that likely to be radium, Nathan?'

He sat down slowly, thinking a moment. 'Cobalt, I'd imagine. You'll find details of it somewhere in that book. Yes, radioactive cobalt it will probably be in Robin's case.'

'What will happen, Nathan?'

'Well, small doses of radiation can stimulate healing. In fact, it's sometimes used in the treatment of ordinary conditions – like inflammations. By special techniques, the radiotherapist will concentrate on the malignant tumour tissue only. This reduces the effects on the peripheral cells.'

'Is there a limit to the amount of the dosage?'

'Yes. The measurement of radiation is the rad, you see. That is the unit of absorption of energy per gram of tissue.' He smiled. 'I'm beginning to sound very technical.'

'That's just what I want you to be, Nathan.'

'Well, the body can tolerate and recover from quite large doses of radiation if only small areas are exposed. But larger doses of acute total body irradiation, such as in the immediate region of an atomic explosion, result in very serious affects.'

'What is likely to be Robin's exposure – or could you even guess?' Only with Nathan could I have pushed so hard; asked the unanswerable and yet been sure of no rebuff.

'I just couldn't attempt to say, Inez. It's not my field. But Robin's in the care of an excellent man. However, let's take me,' he paused, running his hand over his thinning grey hair. 'Now, a dose of about 600 rads would temporarily remove all this – if age hadn't already done so! Normally, in a young man, the hair would regrow in about six weeks. But local exposure of say, about 2500 rads, would probably result in permanent baldness. Of course, that's a very superficial illustration.'

It was late. Nathan was old and looking tired. I stood up. 'Nathan, I can never adequately express my thanks – for everything.'

He touched my arm as he showed me to the door. Spontaneously, I laid my fingers over his. It was a pathematic gesture. So much hyper-charged emotion aching to give expression of gratitude.

'I'm so glad I found you that evening in the mountains at sunset time,' It sounded cloying and sentimental.

But he understood. 'Fate was good to me too that night, Inez,' he responded gently. 'Now remember, I'm always here when you need me. Always.'

That night, I started work on the dictionary, following through relevant sections and cross-references.

I learned that in Africa, breast cancer was lower in rate than any-where else in the world; yet liver cancer was very common there. About forty percent of cancer deaths in Iceland came from stomach malignancies. Rectal cancers were twice as common in Denmark as in Norway.

International statistics; inexplicable at the time when the book had been compiled.

I'd heard a mention of metastasis. This, I discovered ,was a secondary growth. Tumours could metastasize to quite distant locations; and the larger the tumour, the greater the possibility of metastasis. Robin's growths, to date, appeared to be exclusively in the abdominal region.

On then to radium; cobalt. A metallic element of atomic no 27. Cancerous or malignant cells are more responsive to radiation than normal healthy cells. Deep-seated cancers are often treated with supervoltage X-rays by a machine designed to penetrate through to the tumours.

I laid the dictionary aside. There was a relief in knowledge; in understanding a little better.

Nathan's words echoed in my mind 'Now remember, I'm always here when you need me. Always.'

Robin's morning was marked with activity. After breakfast, he was washed. He cleaned his teeth and brushed his hair himself. His dressings were changed.

In the Nurses' Station, Dr Monaghan explained his plans for Robin's treatment. 'The tablets we're giving him are intended to counteract spasms and eliminate griping pain.' He glanced up shyly, then looked away. 'The treatment is designed to shrink the growths. There are probably quite a number of affected lymph glands still active. Now deep ray treatment in the abdominal area nearly always causes discomfort while the treatment lasts. You understand that?'

I nodded silently. He continued. 'Sometimes diarrhoea or vomiting can be a side effect. I'll start Robin with thirty seconds of cobalt, increasing daily. The treatment will take somewhere between a fortnight and a month. And you'll have to remember that he's a very very sick child.'

He let a moment elapse. Then went on. 'A complete cure is not impossible. But it isn't very likely. Not impossible; but highly improbable.'

There was no need for words. No questions to ask. It had been honestly assessed and frankly explained.

'I'll probably give him tablets when he goes home, to keep the affected glands shrivelled up. But whether or not it will spread to other lymph glands, time alone will tell. However, he shouldn't ever again have the pain he has experienced. If the other glands become affected they may show by swellings, not necessarily pain.'

He opened his hands in an expansive gesture, hesitating before he spoke. 'As to the future? Heaven alone knows. But with the help of God, it shouldn't be too bad. We can't attempt to forsee it.'

Incipient relief, like a warm glow, crept over me. The candour, the simplicity of this extraordinary unpretentious man began to banish the festering resentments of the past. The fears of the future. The days of anxiety and anguish might not be over; but nothing could ever again be so harrowing. The fight for Robin's right to die in peace was no longer a solitary war to be waged alone. This quiet doctor really cared, was personally concerned and planning positively for the well-being of a child who had, for months, been almost abandoned to fate.

He saw the tears that blinded my vision. He looked away.

A high-pitched bleep sounded from his pocket. Someone else needed him. 'The next thing we've to do,' he said softly, 'is to get Robin up and moving round again.'

Robin's treatment began that afternoon. He was kitted out in dressing-gown and slippers. A green-coated porter arrived with a wheelchair.

'Why don't you come along with him?' he suggested to me. 'It will give him confidence.'

Robin was pushed along to the Radiotherapy Department. A bright airy hall with small changing cubicles and several X-ray treatment rooms.

A number of radiotherapists were in attendance. Dr Monaghan came over to Robin.

'Feeling okay?' he asked.

Robin was 'screened'. Details were filled in on a treatment sheet; notations of the area to be treated and the dose of cobalt to be administered. The skin was marked with blue outlines.

An attractive radiotherapist, in a trim-fitting white coat, then took Robin into the treatment room. He was lifted on to the table and settled comfortably. It was a sealed room, artificially lighted, with a glass window through which she could watch him.

The over-head X-ray machine was adjusted. Her friendly chat dispelled any apprehension Robin might have had. She placed a pushbell near his hand in case he wanted to call her during treatment.

I followed her out. Robin looked around with interest. The door was closed. She settled herself on a swivel chair at the controls of her plant. She clicked various switches, lights illuminated the dials. Through the window panel, I could see Robin lying quite still. In less than a minute, it was over. Wrapped in his dressing-gown, he was lifted back into the wheelchair.

Dr Monaghan spoke cheerfully. 'That wasn't too bad, now was it, Robin?'

It became a daily adventure. Always, after treatment, he vomited. Like sea-sickness, it was preceded by nausea. Then a single bout of vomiting.

'We'll change the treatment to a morning session,' Dr Monaghan decided. 'That way, when the vomiting is over, he can enjoy his lunch.'

At each meal, Robin helped himself liberally from the menu. Took second portions of whatever he particularly fancied.

Sometimes the resulting pain was eliminated by tablets. Occasionally, an injection was necessary. Speedily, it was given.

Each day he was lifted out to sit in an easy chair by the window. An overture to future mobility.

'How about getting out of doors for a while, Robin?' It was a balmy afternoon. Robin was looking out on the gardens as Dr Monaghan passed room No 12.

Robin was wrapped in blankets with an anorak tucked over his dressing gown. Tremulously, I navigated the wheelchair into the lift, through the swing doors of the Reception area and out into the sunshine.

Robin was ecstatic.

For over an hour, he explored a forgotten world of sunlight, movement and colour. His awareness was heightened from months of sensory deprivation. His responses were intense. The delight in the feel of a whispering breeze on his face. The warmth of sunshine on his skin.

'Look! There are conkers over there,' he cried excitedly.

I found a broken branch of beech. From his wheelchair, he probed the carpet of fallen leaves, turning up the green spikey shells. His weak fingers struggled to prise them open. I helped. Each smooth polished chestnut was added to the pile on his blanketed knees; triumphant proof of his will to live.

It was the first of many wheelchair outings. We roamed the landscaped gardens, followed the stream, meandered by the lake. Limpid golden afternoons. Cloudless azure skies. Autumn came gently that year.

'He's responding extremely well to treatment,' Dr Monaghan gave his verdict. The pain was de-escalating but not yet eliminated. 'Now I want to get him walking again.'

A progressive programme was started. Robin sat, trembling with nerves, on the side of his bed, feet dangling. Gingerly, he lowered his weight. The leg muscles protested painfully at the unaccustomed usage. Then, supported by two nurses, he took a couple of steps. The effort drained him. But day by day, he improved. The faltering movements became more confident.

Finally, he managed to take tiny shuffling steps unaided, gripping the bed for balance.

Robin liked to keep his door open, to watch the occasional activity on the passage.

A dull buzzer sounded from a room nearby. A nurse came quickly.

'I want a cigarette,' a senescent voice complained.

'But you've had over twenty today. You're on your second packet.' she protested.

Robin whispered. 'That patient who's just rung: his sight is failing and someone has to sit with him while he puffs . . .'

'Just one more, nurse,' the quavering voice pleaded. There was the sound of an igniting match.

Robin listened with interest.

'I think that poor old man's mind is slipping a bit,' he commented. 'Sometimes I see him wandering out on the passage and the nurses have to lead him back to bed. He doesn't know where he is. Says he wants to go home. It's sad really.' He concluded with the objective detachment of a child with a lifetime of living ahead.

Later that evening, as he lay watching television, a rumbling noise sounded from his abdomen. There was a glutinous discharge, erupting in gaseous bubbles from the wound. A rancid odour of putrification.

The Night Nurse changed the soiled wet dressings and gave him a tranquilliser.

Next afternoon, I met Dr Monaghan. There was no formality in our talks. I was carrying the goldfish tank from the sluice room where I had changed the water, as he came along Ward P.

'Put that on a trolley in future. It's too heavy for you.' he said, lifting it on to its shelf. 'Now, I want to have a word with you for just a moment. Okay, Robin?'

Robin was happily demolishing a plateful of steak and chips. He showed no particular interest.

Together we moved out of earshot.

'I've had an X-ray done. The treatment has shrivelled up the glands so we've discontinued it. But Robin shouldn't be having so much pain. I think it's from all that muck and infection there. I'm going to get his surgeon to look at him again.'

The grey eyes noted my automatic recoil. The incipient fear that his words generated.

'There's no question of surgery,' he reassured me. 'It's just that he may be able to make suggestions.'

Only my absolute faith in his judgment kept the panic from breaking through.

'Whatever you think best,' I murmured.

He read the terror in my face.

The dispute which had left Bob unemployed all summer was settled by negotiation. He returned to work and a heavy stint of overtime which was financially useful but physically exhausting.

A re-arrangement of the visiting rota was necessary. Robin was co-operative. I came mid-morning; and Bramble Grange provided me with a gratis lunch on a tray, while Robin ate his. My mother relieved me in the early afternoon, and took him on his daily wheelchair outing. When she arrived home, I drove back and spent the evening with Robin until Bob came by bus from the city about 9.30 p.m. Then, when Robin was settled for the night, we left him.

The Staff Sister on Ward P had been away on holidays when Robin was admitted for treatment. She returned early in October – Sr Ryan, a plump jolly little woman with perennial good humour, inexhaustible patience and a silvery chuckling voice. She was a reservoir of courage and kindness. At Bramble Grange, she was an institution. Patients and staff uninhibitedly spoke of her with the affection which she richly merited.

Robin's birthday came. There were cards and presents from friends who had not forgotten him. Gifts, too, from the staff. The cook baked a cake, complete with candles and inscribed in soft icing. Sr Ryan carried it in to No 12. Nine miniature glowing flames. We celebrated; I tried to banish the fear that was throttling me.

Next day, the storm broke.

Mr Verkonnen called. I was not there. Robin was in bed, following his afternoon outing in his wheelchair. My mother waited in the passage while the surgeon examined Robin. Presently he emerged and closed the door.

He said that Robin certainly looked much healthier. His proposition was to move him back to Holy Innocents' for examination. She commented that Robin would not like that. 'His memories, you know, are not very happy ones,' she said.

Dr Monaghan was away for a few days' holiday. My time of Schweikism was over. So was my habit of deference to authority *per se*.

From home that evening, I telephoned Dr Castle, the Senior Consultant Radiotherapist at Bramble Grange. I told him of Mr Verkonnen's visit. I knew Dr Castle by appearance. A big white-maned man; formidable, but with an avuncular manner. He always paused at Robin's door with some jocular remark as he made his Ward Rounds.

He suggested I telephone Mr Verkonnen at his home and explain that we'd prefer Robin to be examined at Bramble Grange. The Theatre would be available at any time that was convenient for Mr Verkonnen.

A surge of nerves made me tremble as Mr Verkonnen responded to my introduction. He explained that if Robin was transferred back to Holy Innocents', he would do an examination under anaesthetic. After this, there would be a consultation. They would talk with us. The pain could be coming from a sinus. Surgery would help this but it could not be done at the examination. It would entail another operation.

His words alerted me, turned time back and opened closed chapters. The ghastly scenario of the past was resurrected.

'Robin is extremely happy in Bramble Grange,' I said quietly. 'Naturally his memories of Holy Innocents' are tarnished by the fact that he underwent surgery there. For him, it's synonymous with pain and distress.'

'Of course,' he agreed readily.

'Would it be feasible for you to do surgery in Bramble Grange, if theatre facilities were made available, as I understand they would be?' I felt I was treading on quicksand.

He replied cogently. No! He could not give the post-operative care he would want to provide. He would not have his usual team of staff, and calling to Bramble Grange to assess Robin's progress would not be easy for him.

I whittled words down to the minimum. 'In effect, does that mean that it *must* be at Holy Innocents', as far as you're concerned, Mr Verkonnen?'

'Yes.' He answered succinctly.

Our parting was amicable.

A little later, Dr Castle's resonant voice boomed down the miles of cable. 'Tomorrow I will look further into Robin's case before making any recommendations or reaching any decisions. Meanwhile, the situation is fluid.'

Bob took time off work next day to talk with Dr Castle. It was decided to combat pain as effectively as possible until Dr Monaghan's return. A couple of days more and he would be back.

I saw the familiar white-coated figure come out of the Nurses' Station. He was carrying a file.

I gulped. Tears of relief stung my eyes.

Dr Monaghan shuffled along towards me. 'I've heard what's been suggested,' he began, suntanned fingers tapping the cardboard. 'I'm not too happy about it. Sometimes these problems ease, given time. It might just be a tiny infection that's causing pain. It might clear up, you see. But, unfortunately, in young people, often special attention is needed.'

In utter weariness, I ran my fingers through my hair. 'What do we do?'

'I'd much prefer it if Robin didn't have surgery,' he said sympathetically. Then he added, 'But I quite see Mr Verkonnen's point of view, if major surgery was involved.' He thought a moment. 'I had hoped to let Robin home for a while, that's if he'd be agreeable to come back here again,' he said.

'There'd be no problem on that score,' I assured him quickly.

'This situation is difficult, you appreciate that? I'd like a few days to think about it. Maybe we could play for time.'

'Of course! We're happy with whatever you decide. We feel that all the progress Robin has made is due to you and to Bramble Grange. That's why we would be extremely reluctant to move him elsewhere. You do understand?'

He nodded. Warm grey eyes lighting the thin face.

And Time proved to be our friend.

Robin was encouraged to select a lighter diet from the menu. Gradually, the frequency of pain diminished, lessened in intensity. Each few
days marked a little progress. Outings in the grounds were preceded
by getting dressed.

I bought new clothes for him. Polo-necked sweaters for warmth as
his shirts hung loosely on his scraggy neck, long trousers to cover the
shrivelled shanks. He started walking alone without support. A wobbling windmill figure, all legs and arms.

'Try taking him home. Just for a short spell in the afternoons,' Dr
Monaghan suggested.

I lifted the featherweight body from the wheelchair on to the
passenger seat of the car. Robin was tense with excitement.

At home he lay on a sofa, rediscovering familiar surroundings.
Billie, slightly shy of this half-stranger, brought him his favourite
books. Helen, with her retarded intelligence, jumped around him.
Robin insisted on holding seven-month-old Michael in his arms. Then
he played a desultory game of chess, in the flicker of firelight. Everything was new and exhilarating again.

He was back in Bramble Grange in time for tea.

The injections were dispensed with. Tablets sufficed now to kill the
pain. Their action was slower but effective.

Robin knew he must be patient. He drew on Herculean reserves of
self-discipline, gave the tablets time to work, cooperating fully.

'Tomorrow you can try taking him home for the night. We'll see
how it goes,' Dr Monaghan said a few days later.

It worked.

Sr Ryan collected a supply of tablets and dressings.

'Drop in on us whenever you are running short,' she said cheerfully,
packing them in a bag.

Nervously, I posed the question. 'From your experience, what do
you think the future might hold, Sister?'

She sat down at her desk, glancing at the laden shelf of coloured
files which told the case histories of her patients on Ward P.

'No one can tell you how or when, you know. It might start with
weakness or vomiting. Probably there'll be very little pain. But every

person differs and no one can tell.'

She looked out at the parklands. A flight of late migrant birds swooped, wheeled, turned south to the horizon. Start of a journey; some would die on the way. Many would reach their haven in the sunshine.

'We've let patients go,' she said slowly, 'and not expected to see them for six months; they might be back in a few weeks. Others don't return for much longer. A few – they never come back at all.'

FIVE

October to June – The Pendulum Months

'I am a pilgrim of the past, making
a journey into the future.'
Pierre Teilhard de Chardin, S.J.

Robin had the resilience of youth. His return home gave him a psychological uplift. The whole disintegrated fabric of family life began to weave together again into something resembling normality.

Many of his first days were spent in bed. Gradually he stretched the range of his activities as his strength returned. His spirits were buoyant though his body was weak. The physical strain on me increased. But there was the compensation of seeing him improve.

Bramble Grange had supplied him with an assortment of tablets, some to counteract the griping pain which occurred after each meal. He also had 5 mg Valium pills – tranquillisers which he took in moderation to induce sleep.

The fumarolic hole in his abdomen occasionally erupted and discharged gaseous bubbles of faecal matter. He dressed the wound himself, carefully opening the sterilised packets, cleaning away the malodorous brown fluid, placing the soiled dressings in a disposal bag for incineration.

I continued to keep a diary of events . . .

On November 5th, Robin had a restless night, troubled by nausea and pain which defied attempts at alleviation. At mid-day, the wound opened and pus poured out. I rang Bramble Grange.

'Bring him down,' Dr Monaghan said promptly. 'I'll arrange a bed for him right away.'

The rain lashed as Bob carried the worn body into the hospital.

The wound was dressed. Dr Monaghan looked in on him. There was a pungent fetid smell in the room. A sedative was ordered. Presently, Robin slept – his skin ashen against the white pillowcase.

'Poor lad. He's exhausted from the whole experience.' Dr Monaghan's vulpine face was soft with concern. He murmured something about a sinus.

The wind bullied the trees outside, shaking the leaves from the sodden branches. Night Sister called on her rounds. She stopped to talk with us. I had always related a sinus to a nasal condition. I asked her about it.

'It's a burrowing ulcer, you could say. It takes the form of a blind tube. Usually pus forms at the blind end and reaches the body surface, as in Robin's case. In this instance, it's abdominal.'

'Will it heal up, do you think, Sister?'

'I couldn't honestly say.' A fresh-air fragrance of Tweed perfume wafted pleasantly from her. 'If it is a sinus and it breaks inside, then it would make him very sick indeed. It could take several days to clear, and there's always the possibility it might recur from time to time.'

Next day, Robin had diarrhoea; but he ate a good dinner.

Dr Monaghan had his own blue-print of priorities. 'I want to get Robin back home as quickly as possible.' He assessed the situation. 'There appears to be seepage from the bowels. This would and will set up infection and sometimes make him feel off-colour. It's not likely to clear up completely but I think we can discharge him tomorrow or the next day. He'll be in and out of here from time to time to have this attended to. But the important thing is to have him based at home.'

Robin was discharged.

It was the same day that Lilian Board flew to Germany on the start of the last lap of her fight against cancer . . .

. . . The newspapers, radio and television bulletins gave it wide coverage. Graphically; too graphically for me. Each report wrenched another drop of pity from my tattered emotions.

Dr Issels' Ringberg Clinic at Rottach-Egern. Walks in snow-covered Bavarian mountains.

Preliminary extraction of two front teeth.

An improvement. No pain.

Shopping sprees to buy snow boots and warm winter clothes.

Tonsillectomy without general anaesthesia. Quick recovery. Family reunion for a holiday weekend.

Complications from Barium tests of three months' previously. Diminishing appetite, drooping morale. Bouts of pain.

Another colostomy-type operation. This one was at Tegernsee. The discovery that her stomach was filled by a massive tumour.

She returned to the Clinic. Resurgence of hope. Weeks of waiting. Lilian, *in absentia*, voted as Sportswoman of the Year.

Cautious medical optimism. If she could hold her own for a fortnight, things might be brighter.

Deterioration in December. One hour's surgery to drain fluid from her abdomen.

Her birthday. Twenty-two years old. A coma. Heart injections and a slight improvement. Then suspected peritonitis. Surgery for stomach blockage.

Christmas Eve. Everything was tried. Oxygen. Injections.

Boxing Day. Her father holding her hand when the pulse stopped. Lilian Board was dead . . .

Christmas came and went for us. It was unlikely that Robin would ever celebrate another. I expunged the past and lived in the present.

New Year's Eve and the golf clubhouse was asparkle with fairy lights. Christmas trees twinkling with tinsel and the tinkle of silver bells. Count down to midnight . . . Four . . . Three . . . Two . . . One . . . Zero! *Auld Lang Syne.* Hands joined. Friends who had helped us through the past year.

Goodbye, Old Year! Goodbye!

'Happy New Year.' My fingers, intertwining in Bob's, clung desperately. May it not be as bad as the year that's ebbed away.

We broke into couples. Kisses. Dancing. Laughter.

Six months of Gothic horror. Horror observed; experienced. The most traumatic through which I had ever lived or would ever wish to live. I had lost faith in religion but not in Man. I had learned to look on fear and death; and spit in the face of both. The spittle of hate but not defeat. I had learned to analyse my terrors and discard the trivia of superfluous anxieties and worries about events over which I had no control.

Home before dawn.

Return to reality. Robin was tossing restlessly.

He had pain that morning. Then around mid-day a violent spasm which contracted his body and forced his knees up to his chin. Disprin and a hot water bottle helped to ease it. But the area between the groin and the genitals twinged with occasional jabs of pain.

Two days later, Robin began to cry. A discharge from the penis had hardened into little crystals and the pressure of passing urine caused soreness. A warm bath and swabbing failed to alleviate it.

He was admitted to Bramble Grange and put to bed. At 1.30 p.m. a young house surgeon started to work on clearing away the murky droplets.

Sr Ryan walked the corridor with me. 'It may just be a pus-like discharge, Mrs Heron.'

'But it could be the augury of further trouble, Sister – yes?'

'It's best to appreciate what's good. Robin has had a respite. He also responds splendidly to treatment. But, you know, it's only palliative. While we can continue to hope, it's wise to realise that it may be short-lived.'

A couple of hours passed. After poulticing and dressing it with ointments, the globules dissolved.

Robin came home again.

Dr Monaghan arranged for a lymphogram test and the following afternoon, I took Robin back to Bramble Grange.

He walked in from the car and we waited in a four-bedded ward. He was very silent. Half-an-hour later, he was wheeled away to Theatre on a stretcher, his hair a blaze of colour on the shiny plastic-encased pillow. I sat on.

A junior Radiotherapist came to the Ward. A man, this time. 'We're having a bit of difficulty,' he explained apologetically. 'It would be best if you called back in a couple of hours.'

Robin was weepy on his return to the ward but an injection made him drowsy.

The Radiotherapist was regretful. 'We've made four efforts to inject into the lymph vessels in the foot. Robin has proved to be one of the ten per cent of cases which cannot be treated in this way. It's due to various complications, the fineness of the vessels, etcetera.' He paused, then continued. 'It would have helped Dr Monaghan by showing just what the condition of the glands currently is; whether or not they're enlarged or irregular in any way. Of course, it couldn't obviate the necessity of treatment for a condition which may, or may not, be deteriorating. Anyway, we'll leave the stitches in his foot for the moment. Removing them will be simple, don't worry.'

We didn't tell Robin that it had all been in vain. At home again, he spoke of it himself.

'I had an injection before the lymphogram test. It knocked out my leg although I could feel the rest of my body. In my leg, there was nothing but a sensation. A jerk, but not pain, as they nicked the skin. I was amazed that I could feel so little.'

Later that night, Nathan telephoned me. His was philosophical. 'Failure to carry out a lymphogram test, owing to the smallness of the vessels, is fairly commonplace. And anyway, the results wouldn't be conclusive. Helpful, yes; but not definitive. It's just as well Robin doesn't know it wasn't successful.'

On January 6, Robin had a routine scheduled check-up with Dr Monaghan. 'I can feel swelling in the abdominal area. I'm going to have a blood count done and an X-ray of the small intestine.'

He glanced at Robin who was dressing himself in the inner surgery after examination. 'He's looking very wan. I'm going to try injections. Chemotherapy. They're very expensive. Now, I believe you mentioned you had family connections with the pharmaceutical trade. I'll give you the name and details of the drugs and you can bring them in to me. That way, it will be easier on you financially.'

I bit my lip to ease the trembling which this man's extraordinary kindness always aroused in me. He noticed it. 'There now,' he murmured. Soft sounds of comfort. 'We'll start with four injections. One weekly.'

He reached for a pad and made a notation in his small neat writing. 'I may possibly give him more. And maybe another course of Deep Ray treatment – probably in conjunction with the injections.'

At Out-patients Department, on January 18, Robin shed his shoes and socks and lay back in a quasi-dental chair. Within minutes the stitches were out. My tension was almost tangible in the clinical atmosphere. The doctor eased the sock over a dressing on Robin's foot.

Gingerly, and limping slightly, Robin walked out to the car.

Two days later, I carried a neat pharmaceutical package of drugs in to Bramble Grange and placed it on Dr Monaghan's desk. He unwrapped the little cardboard cartons and checked the phials before filling a giant-sized syringe.

Robin sat stiff with apprehension.

'Don't look,' I pleaded.

'I want to look,' he muttered aggressively. Dr Monaghan was lost in concentration. He tried both Robin's arms, but the veins wouldn't rise. Despite the warmth of the consulting room, my teeth were chattering.

'I'm having a block and getting nowhere,' he said finally. 'They may be luckier down in Out-patients. Okay, Robin?'

Incredibly, the red head nodded without demur.

The duty doctor was very reassuring, a Staff Nurse helped him. On the second attempt, he emptied the syringe into the vein.

Another massive injection was mainlined into Robin's system a week later. But the response, Dr Monaghan felt, was below par.

'I'm going to try further Deep Ray treatment with Robin. He'll be an out-patient, of course. And I think it would be psychologically beneficial if you could start him back to school. Just a partial return; a few classes, as much as he feels able to comfortably manage.'

The slow and erratic process of rehabilitation began.

A letter arrived for Bob. It came from Mr Verkonnen, enclosing his account for Robin's surgical treatment at Holy Innocents'. It was a courteous note explaining that in view of all the circumstances surrounding Robin's illness and the considerable expense involved, our account to him need not exceed our benefit for the surgery which was payable by the Voluntary Health Insurance Board, to which we were contributors.

It was a considerate and generous gesture. Fortunately, our insurance coverage was almost adequate to meet the bill in full. We made up the small difference from savings.

The account was worded in medical jargon. I could recognise no mention of appendicitis.

(date) Resection of terminal ileum part of cecum

(date) Right hemicolectomy

(date) Labyrinthotomy intestinal obstruction

(fee) £ —————.

The letter ended expressing gladness that, from accounts, Robin was well in himself; and that, if we would like Mr Verkonnen to see him at the Holy Innocents' Clinic, we could phone and make an appointment.

We didn't. For me, Holy Innocents' was a closed chapter. Robin felt the same. One night he spoke of his time there. We were chatting in his bedroom before he settled to sleep.

'You know, once I had an idea of escape. Although I couldn't walk, I knew the French door of my room opened onto a balcony. I thought of sliding down the pole and crawling on my hands and knees to the barbed wire fence. You'd be coming in to sit with me, and maybe you and Dad would see me and take me home. But then I was afraid that if I fell and broke my arm or something, I'd be there longer.' He smiled at the memory. 'It was just an impossible dream.'

The hiatus between the past and the present was too wide to be bridged.

We never telephoned Holy Innocents'.

Deep Ray treatment was given after school hours. It continued through February, several times weekly.

On the final day, Dr Monaghan examined Robin. It seemed an opportune time to mention summer holiday plans.

'We usually rent a house at Lisclahane on the Atlantic coast for the month of June. And Robin's Grannie is anxious that he should visit Lourdes, perhaps at Easter. Frankly, Dr Monaghan, what do you think we should do?'

'Don't think too much about the future, Mrs Heron. Make your plans. Then face each event as it comes. As to Robin's condition, I can't pretend that he has a fifty-fifty chance. Firstly, he has damaged intestines. There could be an obstruction at any time. A lump could grow again. You see, you can give so much Deep Ray treatment and after that, there just isn't any point. It won't do any further good. So go ahead and make your plans.'

It was March when the incredible day came. The day when Robin experienced no pain. He had eaten his regular meals, augmented by snacks. No digestive pain resulted. Nine months, each day marred by suffering. Now, at last, it was over. By degrees, pain began to be the exception rather than the norm.

Robin's strength was percolating back. After school, when the weather was fine, I collected him and Billie straight from their classrooms, and we went fishing.

One afternoon I sat on the river bank desultorily reading, acutely aware of awakening spring around me. There was almost a hint of summer in the shafts of sunlight which touched the silver fur of a pussy-willow.

Robin was casting in the shallows. I watched him; a slightly bent round-shouldered figure beneath the brown quilted anorak. The medical miracle of Deep Ray treatment.

He wandered nearer the waterfall, perilously near. It cascaded down into a seething pool of foam some forty feet below. I almost called out a warning. Almost. Then stopped. Resisted the inclination. A sudden shout might cause him to teeter; to lose his balance; to crash over the edge . . .

. . . Debilitated body, hurtling helplessly. Violent impact as it cleaved its way through the white froth to the still brown waters of the deep cavern beneath. Suffocating lungs forcing it to surface. Struggling. Clawing hands raking frenetically for a hold. A worse fate or a better one than that which lay ahead?

I sat silent. Poised; tense. Didn't call out. Left destiny in the fickle fingers of fortune.

Robin moved. Meandered upstream again.

It was gone. The moment that might have brought a merciful end. It was the first time, the only time since that nightmare night in Holy Innocents', that Euthanasia had crossed my mind.

We packed a lot of living into those weeks. Robin's mental inertia vanished with the stimuli of new experiences and discoveries.

We explored the city's docklands, consulting the newspapers for the arrival and departure of ships. Along the cobbled wharfs we drove to see the merchantmen, the freighters, dredgers and tugs. We watched the scavenging gulls and the wading waterbirds.

When Robin was tired, he recharged his batteries by recuperating for a day in bed.

At the end of March, the suppurating wound burst open. A gargantuan flood emptied itself; festering waste matter drooled out. But by

April a scab had formed and only a neat Band-Aid was necessary to protect the wound from the friction of his clothes.

My mother had great credence in the efficacy of Our Lady of Lourdes. I had none. To transport the suffering from one venue to another; to put them through the atavistic rituals of prayer, blessings, immersion in icy water in the hope of a cure for body or soul, defied logic. If a deity could perform a miracle of healing, it could rationally be done anywhere, anytime, I felt.

My memories of Lourdes were frightening in the context of Robin's trauma. The stricken bodies laid out on stretchers; white-robed bishops with raised monstrances blessing the afflicted. Amplified distorted voices exhorting thousands to prayerful incantations.

No! Lourdes was not for me. I had no faith.

Bob took Robin and Billie to the Shrine with a small group of thirty pilgrims and no invalids. He tried to make it a holiday for them. They stayed in a hotel and deliberately missed out on most of the religious ceremonies which, Bob felt, would prove harrowing for Robin. They made trips on a funicular railway to a mountain summit; trips to the country on a snowy road, walled by banks of ice from an impacted avalanche; and trips to the Roman Fort above the town.

At home, the weather was kind. I dug a hole in the vegetable garden and lined the brown earth with sheets of thick polythene. I filled it with water and placed the goldfish tank in the pool.

Slowly, the fish nosed their way uncertainly into the open waters. Then, feeling the freedom of space, they gained courage. Soon the sinuous golden bodies were flashing across the pond; fins spread wide, exploring the crannies of shade beneath the rocks.

My task done, I straightened up. The water sparkled; diamond crystals of liquid sunlight.

Unwittingly, I had quarried out the pool for the shape, size and dimension of a child's grave.

I shuddered.

Robin returned from Lourdes and was delighted with the fishes' freedom. He headed for the local river with net and jam-jar. 'Look, Mum, I've caught some pinkeens.'

He eased them into the pond. The goldfish accepted them without aggression. One pinkeen developed a fungal growth on his pectoral fin. He died. Within a week, disease had emptied the pool of all life. I buried the six bodies.

One evening, Robin spotted a centipede in the contaminated water. He tried to scoop it up on a shovel. It wriggled and fell, struggling to gain a foothold on the slippery polythene.

Robin put a pebble under it. Gradually he dredged it up. Its minescule legs flayed the air ineffectually. It was dark brown now; the gleaming orange pigment dulled by submersion.

He lifted it out and placed the pebble on the soil. The centipede lay motionless. Then slowly life seeped back into the tiny organs and limbs. It lifted its antennae tentatively and took a few wavering steps.

Robin held his breath. 'Ssssh! Don't make a sound!'

The centipéde, sensing the nearness of the familiar earth, slithered off the pebble and felt the soil beneath its intricate framework of legs. Then it slowly navigated its shaky way to safety.

Robin sighed with relief. 'Well, that's done. At least we've saved one little life.'

Salvation at the hands of the doomed.

It had been a completely happy day for us.

I went to London and stayed with friends who were more than friends to me. The strength eked back into my body, mind and spirit.

One morning, in a large plate-glass window of an Oxford Street store, I caught sight of a reflection. It was a woman; bright, alert, a zest for living in her step and demeanour. I looked again. It was me.

In the eye of the hurricane, there is a quiet area of tranquillity. An illusion of security. Those in the cockpit know that the only way out is through further convulsive turbulence.

But the respite is good. So good.

The holiday I never dreamed would come materialised that June. We motored across Ireland to Lisclahane. It was the Whit weekend; the month stretched ahead of us.

Semi-tropical weather. Halcyon days. Renewed friendships.

The village teacher's son was a fishing enthusiast. At the start of the season he had bought a new boat equipped with echo-sounder. Robin and Billie spent two intoxicating days out on the bay.

'We've ninety feet of water below. Let your lines down.' They did. 'The basking shark feed on cod. The cod follow the pollock; the pollock chase the sprats. You're sure to get something.' The slaughter began . . .

The evening of the second day, I was in the kitchen. Tomatoes blistered under the grill; potatoes fried to a rich golden brown. I heard the threesome come up the road. High-pitched voices shrieking with excitement. They carried their fish . . .

. . . A film frame. Twenty-four per second; frozen forever in memory. Two jubilant boys dancing with delight. The stalwart weather-bronzed figure of the teacher's son.

Billie was holding two great fish, hideously dangling from barbarous hooks. Robin hugged an even bigger one, loosely wrapped in polythene. Scales and sand spilled with a stinking smell over his chest. They stood in bas-relief at the kitchen door, dark silhouettes against a drained blue summer sky . . .

'The fish hadn't a chance.' Billie exclaimed triumphantly. 'They were giving themselves up.'

Robin interpolated. 'We'd a total catch of fifty pollack and eleven mackerel. We gave the mackerel to some people on the quay. We brought these pollack home just to show you!'

The rest had been discarded in litter bins at the harbour.

The butchery made me sick.

Death on a sun-drenched afternoon. As nauseating as a successful shoot when thundering guns leave senseless carnage behind. Maimed and broken feathered bodies fluttering futilely in a struggle to fly.

'Fish don't feel pain,' the teacher's son proffered, recognising my revulsion. An exhausted hypothesis. Unproven.

'Tomorrow, Dad is taking us to Spanish Point for shore fishing. We can cast from the rocks there. The tide will be right in the morning.' Drowsy voices articulated dreams and plans.

When the boys were sleeping, I carried the stiffened bodies of the fish down to the harbour. Rigor mortis had glaciated them into garbage. Great sad silver-black shapes. A double row of serrated teeth. Dark glazed eyes; moonstones, dull yet with deep shadowy depths of light.

I dropped them into the water.

Robin was listless next morning but he took his fishing gear and Bob drove the boys to Spanish Point. Robin's mood deteriorated. His line caught in seaweed. Dejectedly, he retreated to the car and waited for Billie to tire of casting.

The beach was quilted with sun-soaking bodies. It was the Bank Holiday Monday. The crowds irritated him. He grew petulant.

Back at Lisclahane, he rushed into the house and stumbled up the stairs. I found him lying prone on his bed. He was sobbing.

'What's wrong, Robin? Please, you'll have to tell me. Then we can try and rectify it.' Logic worked.

He turned over on his back. His face was smudged with tears.

'It's my tummy. I've had pain all morning and it's getting worse. Not like the digestive pains I used to have . . .'

I gave him Valium to soothe him and a tablet to combat the pain.

Bob telephoned the local doctor. Luckily, he was at home. I told him Robin's medical history. In the bedroom, he gave Robin a cursory examination. Then he drove to his surgery and returned, within minutes, with morphine.

His lined face was grave. 'It would be best if you took him back to Bramble Grange right away.'

'Will we need an ambulance?' There was a tremor in my voice.

'I don't think so. I've given him a shot that should keep him sleepy for about four hours.' He scribbled a few words for Dr Monaghan on a prescription pad, and dispensed with the formality of sealing it in an envelope.

Friends rallied round. Hasty arrangements were made for the care of Billie, Helen and Michael.

Less than an hour later, we were on the road. Bob drove fast. Robin slept. Then about fifty miles from the city, he began to stir – surfacing from the morphine. He moaned and whimpered. By the time Bob pulled into the deserted car park at Bramble Grange, Robin was screaming with pain. It was 8.00 p.m. Thin rays of sunlight warmed the evening. The fragrance of wallflowers scented the air.

I walked beside the stretcher and through the doors of Bramble Grange.

There was an ominous sense of *déja vu.*

SIX

June, July

'...the dreadful martyrdom must run its course...'
W. H. Auden (*Musée des Beaux Arts*)

The Nursing Staff were on duty in full strength. Just as we reached the Ward Station, Robin began to vomit. He was put to bed in No 10. Ward P. The House Surgeon examined him while the crucifying spasms of pain wracked him. Two injections were given.

Dr Monaghan was contacted by telephone. He gave instructions.

A Ryle's tube was inserted to stop the vomiting and to draw off the build-up of fluid in the stomach.

A drip was linked into his vein. 'It includes an antibiotic,' Night Sister explained.

I sat there, feeling the awful ineffectiveness of my position.

The beginning of the end. I had lost the opportunity of letting him die that spring day at the waterfall. Even a deliberate overdose of sleeping tablets, washed down with alcohol. That would have done it, though it might have earned me a life sentence for infanticide. Anything, anything to have obviated this . . .

Dr Monaghan came in – unfamiliar in sports clothes, a paisley patterned cravat tucked into the neck of his shirt.

He made his points succinctly. 'I've called the radiographer. She'll be here soon. Now, as I understand it, if there is surgery involved you would want the job done here at Bramble Grange. I'm going to try and contact Mr Jeff McMahon. He'll have a look at Robin. He's a Consultant at St Victor's,' he added, 'but he's also one of our visiting surgeons.'

It was an eminent name in medical circles.

The radiographer arrived, golf clubs and a caddy car crammed in the back of her car. She walked briskly up the path and shortly came into No 10.

'It will be reassuring for Robin to have you along with us,' she suggested. His bed was pushed down to Diagnostic X-ray. Two photographic plates.

I traipsed back behind them to Robin's room. Blue and gold wallpaper. The view from the window was the same as from that which he'd previously occupied.

He had ricocheted back in time to a maze of suffering. 'I want to die. Please kill me someone or I'll commit suicide. My life is useless. It's only bloody pain and misery, almost always. I'll never be free of it. Never! That damn God is cruel to create me for this.'

I shared his feelings.

A taxi pulled into the car park and a man stepped out. Within minutes Dr Monaghan was introducing us.

'This is Mr McMahon.'

Jeff McMahon. A pleasant man of medium height, late forties. He had a firm handshake. His eyes dominated his otherwise undistinguished face: tawny amber eyes flecked with brown, keenly intelligent and mesmerically attractive.

The anaesthetist came in hurriedly. He was wearing a blue T-shirt. Finally, the Theatre Sister arrived in a coupé.

The team was complete.

At midnight, Robin was wheeled away to Theatre. We left his empty room. Presently a nurse brought tea and sandwiches to the sitting room where we kept vigil.

Desultory comments. The empathy of silence. A branch brushed against the window, a golden cascade of laburnum. Indigo black night sky.

Footsteps on the passage. My body tensed. If Robin were still alive, there would be the full paraphernalia of surgery. The mobile stretcher. Drip stands. A mêlée of nurses.

The echo of footsteps.

Dr Monaghan came in alone. Two hours had passed since Robin was trundled away. Bob stood up expectantly.

Dr Monaghan's soft voice was almost jubilant. 'There were adhesions, leaks, obstructions. But no tumours.'

'You mean, you mean the cancerous lumps haven't grown again?' It seemed incredible.

He confirmed it. 'No. Nothing but the sort of problems one can expect after serious surgery such as Robin had in the past.'

Fifteen minutes later, Robin was back in No 10.

At home, I took a sleeping tablet.

The telephone rang at 5.00 a.m. Bob scrambled downstairs. Through a barbituric haze, I heard his terse replies. 'Yes. I'll come right away.'

My feet touched the carpet unsteadily. A soft-shoe shuffle of steps. Bob gently guided me back to bed and pulled the blankets over my shoulders.

'No. You can't walk – let alone go through with this. Just go back to sleep.'

'But what's happening?' Already the sedative was reclaiming me.

'Night Sister says Robin isn't so good. He's fluctuating up and down. She feels he could easily go in a down period.'

Bob went out into the early light of sunrise. Dreamily I heard the car engine rev, then fade away.

. . . *Please Robin, let go. Just let go; let go* . . .

Bob woke me. He had brought up breakfast on a tray. I was instantly alert. 'Well?'

'It's all right.' A jejune weariness was in his voice. 'I just sat with him for a couple of hours. Occasionally they gave him oxygen. Just to make things easier for him, they said.'

In the pet shop, they netted two goldfish and freed them into the tank I had brought. Robin watched as I placed it on the shelf and refurnished the room with his personal treasures.

'I'm terribly sorry . . . can't talk very well . . . strain . . . terribly sorry.'

The oxygen cylinder with mask equipment stood at the ready. A Ryle's tube from his stomach coiled down his nostrils, secured to his hair by a kirby grip.

It slipped up and out during the day, and had to be reinserted. 'Swallow as if you're taking a big glass of water.'

He struggled to cooperate.

A blood transfusion fed into his vein.

I glanced through the pile of charts and forms. Blood pressure and temperature regularly noted. His abdomen was slightly distended.

Mr McMahon called.

Next morning's telephone call report: 'Condition unchanged.'

But Robin looked better. His hair had been combed, his hands washed. The sheets were fresh and the adjustable bed had been raised on a ladder-structure. The charts were written up every thirty minutes. '*Oral intake – nil*'. A saline drip replaced the blood transfusion.

That night he asked for a bedpan. His bowels moved. The effort brought tiny crystals of sweat to his forehead.

A couple of days passed. I explained our holiday predicament to Sr Ryan.

'Would it be safe for Bob to leave for Lisclahane? Our other children are parked out with friends there but we can't exploit their kindness indefinitely.'

She was in the Nurses' Station. She pushed away her files. 'I think it would be best to wait a few days longer, Mrs Heron. Some people are in the clear after three or four days. With others, it can be a week or more. It's hard to say.'

That afternoon, the theatre gown was removed. Already Robin's body was wasting. A pulse throbbed wildly in his throat . . .

. . . Outside, a small boy had been wheeled in a chair to sit under the trees. Yellow shirt, blue blazer; partially shaven head. Two cabbage butterflies fluttered by. The boy watched them; dizzy dancers in a sun-soaked minuet. A young male nursing orderly tucked a rug around the diminuitive body. Then he pushed the chair for a little walk and parked it again beneath the trees.

Bewildered child; separated from home, friends, family.

His battered teddy-bear fell from his blanketed lap on to the grass. An old man, sitting on a fallen tree trunk, saw the predicament. He rose stiffly, ambled across the lawn, and handed the toy back to the motionless child. The little boy clutched it, cradling it tightly in his arms . . .

In No 10, the drip hissed with a rhythmic buzz and a flurry of bubbles danced surfacewards from the green needle inserted into the bottom of the jar.

Dr Monaghan came in quietly. Shaken out of reverie, I stood up.

'Don't stir,' he waved me down. 'I'm not important. Not a surgeon or anything.'

His hand rested on Robin's stomach. Robin shivered. 'Oh! It's cold!'

'There, don't worry about that. You've had so much pulling around that you're very sensitive. It's bound to happen. But your tummy's not distended any more; and as your bowels have moved, you should be more comfortable soon.'

He came over to the window and spoke in an undertone. 'I was very worried that first night after surgery. That's why we called you. But Robin seems to be coming on nicely now.'

Mr McMahon called next afternoon. The abdominal wound was oozing. I waited in the sitting room. Presently he came in to speak with me.

His manner was didactic but without any condescension. The beautiful eyes held mine. Beauty was a quality I appreciated in a world of much ugliness.

'Robin has a slight infection in that wound. It's regrettable but not unusual. Two of those stitches can be taken out now. And I'm starting him off on sips of water. One ounce each hour.'

A nurse had placed a meshed dressing pad over the wound, a sterilised tweezers in her hand. Robin's head moved more easily on the pillow.

'Look, Mum! The tube's gone. The Ryle's tube. Mr McMahon took it out himself. He really is an expert. Just told me what he was going to do. Then he whipped it out. I hardly noticed it.'

I felt an upsurgence of gratitude. An appreciation of this frank competent surgeon. It was a feeling that was to grow to admiration and respect for the man himself.

The days moved on.

Progress.

The drip was removed. Robin started to drink milk and tea. Three injections daily. Previously they had been inserted in the drip. His blistered lips looked garish, pigmented with gentian violet and an emollient ointment to avoid cracking.

He was given Complan. 'It's thick, like porridge,' he pronounced, 'but it's not too bad.'

Again, Mr McMahon briefed me. 'I want Robin to have a high protein diet. It's essential for him. That's where you can help. Try and encourage him to take it. Also, he'll be getting two suppositories daily. That should ease things for him.'

Bob returned to Lisclahane. My mother joined me on the visiting roster. Over a week had passed since surgery. Robin began to be fractious and distressed.

His stomach gurgled and erupted gases. 'It's leaking a lot now and it's terribly sore. Like wind pains in my tummy.'

He ate a little minutely minced meat.

A stormy evening. Thundery vermilion clouds. Shafts of golden light touched the beeches. A starling flew past on a late-night sortie. A swish of black and white splotched against the window.

'It's not diarrhoea,' Robin diagnosed laconically. 'It's the normal consistency for a bird.'

I was suddenly aware of how adult he had become. How, through twelve months of illness, he had forfeited much of childhood.

Next morning, Dr Monaghan telephoned. It was early.

'We have to operate again,' he said. Hope plummeted down into despair. He went on. 'I can't underplay the seriousness of this, Mrs Heron. There has been extensive damage to the intestines from the growths of last year; and from surgery and radium. It appears that the leaking is causing the intestines to adhere to the abdominal wall. To leave Robin in this condition any longer would be very unwise. Mr McMahon will operate this morning – with your permission.'

Jesus! Not again! I hesitated momentarily. But there was no real quandary. My absolute faith in these two men conquered my qualms.

I verbalised my consent.

A trunk call to Lisclahane. I told Bob.

It was ten days since Robin's fourth operation.

The journey from Alpha to Omega had begun.

No 10 was deserted. Outside Robin's door his furniture and trolley stood. *101 Dalmatians* lay, earmarked, where he had left it the previous night. Pencil, notebooks: scribbled observations in a childish hand recorded the activities of the magpies which were nesting in a beech tree. An empty urinal, covered by a polythene cloth, lay on its side. The floor had been washed with disinfectant. Patches of damp dried in the breeze from the open window.

Sr Ryan carried in a chair. A nurse brought mid-morning tea.

'Robin's gone about ten minutes,' Sr Ryan said gently.

'Everything is so calm.' It sounded fatuous. My bowels felt loose with fear.

'You wouldn't have thought so if you were here an hour ago when we were getting him ready for surgery, Mrs Heron.' The warm silver voice.

Outside, sparrows tumbled busily in a dustbath under the crimson floribundae. A gardener kick-started a motor mower. It purred comfortingly, weaving symmetric patterns on the lawn. Sunshine transformed tiny microcosms of dust into shining airborne beauty.

Time drifted by . . .

I heard the tinkle of the lunch trolley. A dinner tray was brought to me and Sr Ryan looked in.

'Try to eat now, Mrs Heron. And don't worry. The time lapse is no indication of the situation, or Robin's condition. They mightn't have started surgery right away, you know.'

Another hour passed. She came back.

'They've just phoned from Theatre. Robin is coming over now.'

'Can I stay here, please? I won't be intrusive, Sister, I promise.'

'Of course, you can,' she smiled warmly. 'You've extraordinary courage.'

The depth of that courage was quickly tested. I'm not squeamish. But I had never before seen the corollaries of major surgery. It was a grisly initiation.

Two porters pushed Robin's bed into position. A knot of nurses moved around, each efficiently tending their respective jobs.

'. . . repairs to fistulas . . .' Whispered words.

It was three hours since he had left for Theatre. To my untutored eyes, it looked as if he had come from an abattoir. Blood-soaked sheets. Blood smears on boney arms. Glutinous scummed mouth lolling open. Rolling glazed eyes.

Robin's weak whimpering. 'Help . . . Oh! help . . .' Sudden vomiting. Green bile juice. Lumpy curds in the chrome kidney dish. Abdominal wound pouring fluid and serum.

Expertly, they changed the sheets. A nurse beckoned me over to the bed. 'Take his hand. He's just coming round from the anaesthetic.'

Febrile moaning. 'Pain . . . I've pain in my tummy . . . my chest.'

Icy cold fingers. Blood pressure and pulse check.

'Hold my hand. Just hold my hand. I'm dying . . .'

The drip stand was shifted into position. A blue needle linked it to his vein. A tube drained from the abdominal hole.

Someone closed the venetian blinds to the light, and tidied up the stethoscope and charts on the window ledge. *'Pulse rate 1.30: 1.52.'*

The House Surgeon came in. *'Dr Hunter'* his lapel brooch identified him. I trailed after him to the passage as he left, but he made no attempt to sidle away.

'You're Robin's mother?' He was small, chubby and curly-haired. A charismatic smile that, I later learned, reflected his personality, lit his plump face.

I nodded assent. 'How is he?'

'Mr McMahon found a number of fistulas which he repaired.'

'Fistulas?'

No evasions. 'They're wounds or ulcers causing an abnormal passage between two surfaces; to the skin or to the lining of any hollow organ.' He hesitated. 'We've given him something now. So he'll be sleepy for a while.'

'It's serious, isn't it?' There had been no mention of cancerous growths.

'Well, you know, of course, what's wrong with Robin, Mrs Heron. But Mr McMahon will be back to see him tonight. You could have a word with him then.'

Through stinging unshed tears, I spoke steadily. 'I'll do that. And – thanks for your honesty.'

I was dozing in the sitting room when Bob arrived. He had closed up the house at Lisclahane and brought the children home.

As we prepared to leave, I filled him in on the day.

'You're looking dreadfully washed out,' he said with concern. 'I think you should drop in to Nathan on the way home. Maybe have a check-up.'

For some days I had been feeling niggling chest pains. Not the familiar fibrositic darts that I often experienced in cold winter weather.

Nathan went through the routine procedures. Heart. Blood pressure. Then he sat down.

'You're constitutionally as sound as a girl of twenty. What age are you now, Inez?'

'Thirty-six.'

'Your heart's fine. No murmur; nothing. Blood pressure; excellent. Couldn't be better. The chest pains are probably caused by tension.

I'll give you some more tranquillisers. They should help. Don't be afraid to use them. You've been through a harrowing time.'

His solicitude made me expansive. I told him of Robin's operation. 'So the future doesn't look so bright, does it, Nathan?'

His face was concerned. 'Repairs to fistulas? Well, it could mean possible danger. Look, you will keep in touch with me, won't you? I'm here any time, day or night. You'll do that, yes?'

The unshed tears spilled over in a release of stress.

'There, there. It's good to cry sometimes.' He laid his hand on my shoulder and offered me a large white handkerchief.

Nurse Gilligan was on Night Duty. She was a busy homely girl with thick pebble glasses. Her neatly-rounded derrière was encased in a rose-patterned pantie-girdle beneath her white nylon tailored uniform. She was naturally gregarious. She also was one of the kindest nurses I was ever to meet.

Robin slept sporadically.

Twilight brought rain. It lashed the windows and drenched the trees.

'Robin's very sick, you know,' she said. 'Anything could happen. His pulse is raggedy; jumping about. Poor wee lad. He's been through much more than one human should have to bear.'

His breathing was heavy. Wheezing with each inhalation.

'His chest is full of phlegm. I could hear it at the far end of the passage. I'm going to try and clear it a little.'

Each breath sounded like a death-rattle. She propped him up against her body, holding his hand reassuringly.

'Oh God! . . . I'm suffering . . . suffering . . .' Mucous-filmed mouth.

'I can't give you a drink, Robin. But I've an ice cube here. Just slither it round in your mouth and spit it into this dish.'

He coughed. A knob of sputum belched out. 'Don't try to cough if it's too sore.'

Another barking clearance. With his body's reflex recoil, the drip needle slipped out of the vein.

Nurse Gilligan telephoned Dr Hunter. She was worried.

'If we could rig that drip up again, it might help. Sometimes it gives a bit of a lift. Sort of evens things out.'

She gave him an injection and he fell asleep. Deep stentorian breathing.

At 10.30 p.m., Mr McMahon called. He felt Robin's pulse and touched his abdomen.

'That drip will have to go in again. And a Ryle's tube to keep the stomach clear.' It was twelve hours since he had scrubbed down for surgery. He must have felt as weary as I did. Deliberately, I denied the impulse to scavenge for an impossible prognosis.

The path to the car park was peppered with cigarette ends and dead matches. Stubbed nicotine, quenched out in deference to the threshold of a cancer hospital. The butts lay like trampled canine excreta, saturated by the rain.

In the rhododendron hedge, a blackbird stirred and chirruped uneasily.

Muted bugle call. Taps.

The wailing of police sirens; soaring strings of *Tales from the Vienna Woods*; tolling clock tower chimes; tramping Gestapo boots, heavy, menacing . . .

Robin protested. A television channel was screening *The Diary of Anne Frank*. I had studied the evening's viewing with Robin and lured him away from it. Gruelling epic of cruel inhumanity.

But the soundtrack from Room No 11 intruded relentlessly through the walls. Robin became more embittered. I tried to placate him, though it was also frazzling my nerves.

'Maybe she's a little deaf and she can't hear otherwise,' I feebly suggested.

'Well, she's deafening me, too. Nasty selfish witch!'

For almost two hours it went on and on; interspersed with advertising jingles. I ached to ask a nurse to suggest that the accoustic level be lowered a little. But somehow I distracted Robin and finally it faded to its inevitable close.

Next day, I was glad of my restraint. For the patient in No 11 was Molly Cullen . . .

Anne Frank's first diary entry was written on Sunday, 14th June, 1942. The day, date and month on which, several decades later, Robin had first been admitted to Holy Innocents'.

Anne Frank died at Bergen-Belsen when she was fifteen.

Molly Cullen died, aged fifteen . . .

The vein in Robin's hand was protesting. The drip was inserted in his foot and a protective cage placed over it. His dressings were being changed when I arrived. I waited in the sitting room.

A tall svelte woman was there; very chic in well-tailored slacks and cashmere sweater.

'Your little boy, how's he doing?' she asked.

'He fluctuates. It's a lymphosarcoma.' I opened the morning newspaper, reluctant to become embroiled in discussion.

'Life is so competitive nowadays,' she mused. 'There just isn't room for the handicapped, is there?'

She had convinced herself. The disabilities of the body; the boundless possibilities for a fertile mind. Even a subnormal brain like Helen's could allow an enjoyment of life, in its limited way, given a favourable environment.

She explained that they were waiting for Molly to die. Her face was quite composed, the disciplined control of one who has come to terms with death. Any reply from me would have been trite.

Molly had secondary cancer now, she said. It had started last summer with a lump on her shoulder. She had surgery. She knew it was cancer and spoke about it quite naturally. But she didn't know it was a killer.

I ached for the voice to stop. No more vicarious suffering. Please don't go on!

But she continued. Molly's lungs were now affected. At first the secondary complications had seemed like pleurisy. But now they knew the truth.

A lone swallow played solitaire in the blue sky.

'Her temperature is 103. If it stays up, she'll go quickly – in weeks, perhaps a month. We're taking her home tomorrow.'

I felt her looking at me. Directly at me. 'What age is your son?'

'Robin's nine. Eight when this started.'

'They become more your friends than your children, don't they? Molly's like a sister to me now. She's the eldest of our girls.'

A nurse knocked at the door. 'We've finished with Robin, Mrs Heron. You can go in whenever you like.'

I made my ignoble escape, feeling a guilt at my own inability to offer solace. But words would have been a profanity.

I saw Molly Cullen just once. It was the next day; her departure day. Great brown eyes in a pallid face. A cloud of black hair frothed around her neck. She smiled shyly from her open door.

The poignancy of two stricken young lives.

Anne Frank of Amsterdam – death's victim of genocide.

Molly Cullen of Bramble Grange – death's victim of disease.

A few weeks later, her death notice appeared in the local newspapers. She died at home. Requiem for Molly Cullen.

A week of progress. The yellow drip trailed to Robin's foot. '*Sodium Chloride and Dextrose*', the label on the jar read.

'They've shortened the drain from my stomach and taken out a stitch from the wound,' Robin said.

Mr McMahon commented. 'He's coming on. We'll keep our fingers crossed.'

I probed further with Sr Ryan. 'Guarded optimism is the best way to look at it, Mrs Heron.'

'But, Sister, what can go wrong?'

As always, she was patient. 'Well, internally, quite a lot of things. But it's best not to think too much about them. Actually, he looks much better than after the previous operation. About a week more, and I think we can begin to feel safer.'

Jeff McMahon discussed his plans with Robin. 'Your bowels are doing nicely. They're working and the wind is passing through. Now, naturally, they can't move with nothing inside you. I want you to take some glucose and water orally. And I'm going to take a blood sample.'

A few more days and the stomach drain was removed. Robin was dressed in fresh green pyjamas.

'I had a very good night. But the drip leg gets locked in position. It takes nearly half-an-hour of massage to get it normal again.'

Bread and butter; milk and tea. The drip was taken out and the stitch holding it removed.

A fuller diet. 'Fish or chicken today, Robin?'

A bluebottle buzzed around the room, careering crazily in a whirl of activity; its pregnant body irridescent green with unborn life.

'What sort of fish, nurse?'

'Well, it might be jellyfish – or starfish!'

Robin laughed. A forgotten sound. He settled for steamed cod.

Under the canopy of trees, a boy and girl walked together, as close as his crutches permitted. They came from the shade into the sunshine and sat down on a sloping bank of the lawn, involuntarily moving apart from the other patients.

Casually, she picked daisies. Her fingers wove them into a chain. He leaned forward as she draped it round his neck. Her mouth lingered on his cheek. His scalp was marked by tufted hair and patches of bald skin. She took his hand. Their fingers clasped.

He was about twenty-four. His bed was beside the window of the ground floor ward. In the evening, it was a mecca for visitors; boys and girls of his own age. But this relationship was different: personal, private, precious.

He turned his face to hers. Smiles, words. The intimacy of shared laughter. This moment was theirs for the living. Dappled sunlight played on warm skin that by winter might be decomposing in the inhospitable damp of earth.

It was some time before I saw him again. Only the thinning patches of hair identified him. He was wasted. Ice-white skin, translucent on his prematurely worn face. He had been lifted from a wheelchair and laid on a rug on the grass. His foot kicked patterns on the gravelled path beside him.

When the Allied Forces liberated one of the concentration camps, they placed the living dead in rows outside the huts. There was nothing more to be done for bodies too far gone for a resurgence of life. Bodies laid out in sunlight. Bodies waiting to die . . .

Next night, Robin vomited. Nurse Gilligan explained the medical dilemma. 'The problem is to try and get the body to absorb food and not to aspirate him immediately after intake. As against this, he may vomit if the stomach can't cope with it. We want to get the digestive system working again. That's why we're reluctant to return him to the drip. It's a problem stage, if you like. And we can't estimate how quickly it may be overcome.'

Jeff McMahon returned late that night. He spent some time with Robin; then spoke to me.

'The wound is infected. Probably an abscess. I'll have a swab taken tomorrow.'

'So the situation is still serious?' Like a tenacious terrier, I tried to shake out more information.

The tawny amber eyes assessed how much I could take. Then he replied. 'It could be. There's a danger that the perfectly good pieces of gut which I sewed together may not be knitting properly. If another fistula is forming, there's absolutely nothing surgery can do now. About three days – say, seventy-two hours – should certainly tell. But, you know, Robin should be coming along better than this.'

The abscess burst next morning. A swab was taken. At lunchtime, Jeff McMahon came back.

I was jubilant but he was pragmatic. His fingers fiddled with the cord of the venetian blind.

'We may be lucky, touch wood.' His hand rested briefly on the window frame. 'That infectious matter is coming out. Now, again, I want you to try and get high protein foods into him. They'll help the healing process. Complan, Bovril, soup, minced chicken. Do your best, won't you?'

Robin's face was growing tiny and pinched again. Big twilight-grey wise eyes. An occasional fleeting smile. Pulse 160: 168: 160: 160: 160: 160: 168. It meant nothing to me.

The pain re-erupted. Vomiting became more frequent. The drain was reinserted in his stomach.

The last day of June passed.

'Keep the arm straight, Robin.' Dr Hunter took a blood sample. 'Am I hurting you?'

'No. It's just that I'm scared stiff.'

'There. It's finished now. You're very brave.'

'I'm not brave. Not brave at all,' Robin quavered. It was a heroism bought through endurance.

Muzzy days, fluctuating between fair and bad for Robin. 'Look at me. I'm in dreadful condition. I don't know what's wrong with me.

Sometimes I feel as if I can hardly see or hear. Yet I know you're in the room.'

He was given an enema of olive oil. The veins in his feet collapsed and the drip fluid seeped into the tissue.

'We'll see how well he can tolerate food,' Sr Ryan said.

Chicken. His system revolted. Vomiting. Panic. Aspiration.

'Please, please don't do that!' He begged in agitation.

She reasoned with him. 'It's to prevent the vomiting, Robin.'

'But when you aspirate air, I feel sick. I just know there must be something really wrong with me.'

Later Sr Ryan said sadly. 'He's so intelligent; so mature. He's almost too aware.'

His ankles were swathed in gamgee bandages to ease the friction of pressure from the mattress. Freshly washed and with hair combed, he looked frail. By evening, he looked moribund. Hair spiked with sweat; head drooping on bony concave chest. The rib-frame was a chiselled sculpture. He was propped up on three pillows. A polythene anti-soil sheet lay beneath the rawing red skin of the pelvis. A great gamgee pad covered the surgical wound.

His face contorted, fingers tensed into clawlike fists. Then he relaxed again. 'I can't seem to concentrate any more. Even on the birds outside. But I hear them in the morning. Very early. They're comforting. They're up and about and it almost stops me feeling lonely.'

Off to Theatre for reinsertion of the drip. 'We'll give him sedation before he goes.'

It was evening, but two of the day nurses stayed on late to be with him. I thanked them. 'You're so dedicated. You elevate your work to a vocation rather than just a job.' The language sounded archaic.

They waived it aside. 'Well, Robin knows us. It helps him to have familiar faces with him at a time like this.'

Robin returned with a splint on his leg, the drip feeding into the groin.

Jeff McMahon spoke with Bob on the telephone. 'My worst fears have been confirmed. Another fistula has formed.'

'And so?'

'There is no immediate problem of maintaining Robin at his present level on the drip plus oral protein intake. But the "bug" which causes the fistulas is not responding to antibiotics. We have to depend now on Robin's own antibodies and resistance to it. If he can fight it, well – it should heal up within a fortnight. That is, a fortnight should tell if it is going to heal.'

'What about surgery?' Bob was hobbling himself to any foothold of hope.

'There is absolutely nothing else surgery can do.'

'Mr McMahon, if it doesn't heal, how long can we think in terms of?' Bob prompted an answer from the silent phone. 'Six months? Nine months?'

The reply came firmly. 'It's unlikely to be as long as that.'

There had been references before to infection. But never a 'bug'. This was something different. Viruses; bacteria; bugs?

I delved into Nathan's dictionary before I telephoned him. A virus, I discovered, was a very small form of life, a borderline between living and non-living matter. It was the smallest microbe, or micro-organism, and could not be seen without a microscope. Bacteria came slightly higher up the scale; somewhere between the simple types of vegetable life like fungi and animal life.

Nathan came to my rescue.

'What do you think Mr McMahon meant by a "bug", Nathan?'

'Well, it's hardly a medical definition, Inez. In America, it's applied to any small insect or even a disease-germ. Jeff McMahon probably used it loosely to identify something which is causing infection. Something harmful which establishes itself and multiplies.'

I transmitted the details of Robin's condition. The drip had slipped from the groin. The needle had been reinserted into his hand. A thick milky liquid now fed into the vein: *Intralipid*.

Nathan thought. Then he said, 'As long as something comes from the stomach drain into the Meredith bag – that's the plastic bag that's clipped to the bedstead – well, it's a good thing. It indicates that some small amount of nourishment is being digested and the excess wastage is coming out. At least it's not loose in the abdominal cavity and seeping into the system.'

'And the enemas, Nathan?'

'Well, they'd be clearing away any residue which might be lying around in the intestines.'

'Oh Nathan! How can all this ever improve?' My dejection voiced itself.

'Now, Inez, years ago inflammation of the peritoneum was very serious. Particularly in small children, or indeed in adults. But today, with antibiotics, it can be cured.'

I knew something of the peritoneum. The very thin membrane – vaguely like a film of polythene in texture – which functioned to cover many of the organs in the abdomen, and the abdominal wall itself. When it became inflamed or abscesses formed, seepage could occur. But its indigenous healing powers were good, and once it started to heal, it could become perfectly healthy again.

Nathan was speaking. 'The longer Robin lasts and the more resistance his body can build up – well, the better his chances. But it *is* a real problem. The seepage, you see, increases the toxin in his system.'

I mentioned the blood samples that had been taken.

'Yes,' Nathan said, ruminatively, 'they give a very good panoramic picture of a patient's progress or deterioration. His condition generally, you could say.'

From his dictionary, I'd some knowledge of blood counts. The measure of the number of cells to the cubic millimetre of blood. In diagnosis, there were literally hundreds of different tests. But, basically, there were three main groups. Haematology which gave clues to haemoglobin, clot formation, and condition of cells, etcetera. Then there was blood chemistry; tests which reflected chemical functions throughout the body – sugar, perhaps relating to the pancreas. That would be an indication of diabetes; or various enzymes showing malfunctions of bone, liver, muscles and such like. Finally, there was microbiology. Many types of infection could be identified this way: through immunity, or antibodies, as evidence; or the actual detection of microbes, say malaria or typhoid.

I laboured it further, confident of his endless patience.

'From what I've told you, Nathan, how do you view Robin's chances?'

There was no hesitancy. 'I'll be honest with you. You must be realistic, Inez. It's not by any means rosy with so many adverse factors involved. But it's not irrational to reason that the longer Robin lasts and is bright and alert, the better the indications that his resistance to peritonitis is building-up. However, on the debit side, I can't guess what these blood tests are revealing. And the vomiting – that's not good.'

Barren harvest of hope.

'Most of Robin's intake is coming straight back through the tube. We'll have to keep him on the drip,' Sr Ryan told me. 'We've ordered blood for him. Two units. That should help.'

At lunchtime, a grey van pulled into the car park, a pelican ensignia emblazoned on its side. A smartly-uniformed driver carried a wire crate of white polythene jars into the hospital. He came out again with a load of cardboard boxes and a receipt book.

Robin had a sleepy afternoon. Dr Hunter explained the reason. 'He's been very fretful so we're keeping him sedated. I'm alternating the I.V. feeding, as you've probably noticed, and I've put a drain into the wound. That avoids the necessity of constantly changing the pad. To-night, we'll start the blood transfusion.' He crossed his fingers. 'We can only hope for the best. The general outlook isn't bright, but he seems to be holding his own.'

Later, Sr Ryan changed the dressing and removed the stomach drain. She placed the soiled wastage in a carton.

'We want to send it to Pathology for investigation,' she said vaguely.

That night, a blood transfusion was linked to the vein. A narrow tube carried the dark ruby fluid. The package of plasma was garnet red. A slender wormlike thread dangled, uncoiling along the sheets, feeding into the groin.

I carried the fish tank to the sluice room. Nurse Gilligan was emptying some wilted flowers into a refuse sack. She rinsed out the vase and wiped it carefully, polishing the rim.

I put the fish through their ablutions. We made desultory conversation. It was a dull heavy evening.

She pushed the withered blooms further into the sack and fidgeted with the vase, seemingly reluctant to leave. Then, at the door she paused and turned back.

'Have they said anything to you about the diagnosis?' she asked haltingly.

'In Robin's case?' I stopped, an artificial fern poised in my hand. 'It's a lymphosarcoma. That's what they said at Holy Innocents' . . .'

The words tapered off under her searching look. She closed the door.

What's this all about? Doctors didn't make mistakes. Not those sort of mistakes. Surgeons; pathologists. They had all confirmed it. I had illicitly seen the words. Read them myself: 'Massive growth on back abdominal wall'. Oriel Verkonnen's beautiful bowed head; 'I'd say less than a week to live.' Less than a week to live. Oriel Verkonnen; an eminent name.

'I mean, well – what do you mean? What about the diagnosis?' The sounds stuttered out.

She was silent.

'If it wasn't a lymphosarcoma, just what could it be? Is it not a cancer at all?'

Again the hesitation. The eyes behind the pebble glasses veiled uncertainty. *Christ! What's coming now?* I had to find out. I plunged on, inviting her confidence. 'Mr McMahon did refer to a "bug". But we thought it was some infection. Something in conjunction with the cancer. Is it something else?'

There is no premonition. No predeliction of the moment that proceeds a whole new dimension of horror. One is stumbling along an uneven rocky path. One knows the final destination. And suddenly there's an abyss. A black chasm . . .

I waited. Poised on a *cris de nerfs.*

She spoke professionally, with more assurance. 'If it had been a lymphosarcoma, there would have been metastasis – migration to other areas. Multiple growths. It's almost impossible that Robin could have survived these last months without further major eruptions.'

'The doctors said . . .' I interjected.

'Doctors don't know everything, Mrs Heron. Not by a long chalk.'

Now in terror I was clinging to the awful life-line of cancer. 'But, Nurse, Robin *did* have growths. They were discovered in Holy Innocents'. Treated here last year with cobalt. Treated again at Outpatients in February. Deep Ray therapy.'

People make mistakes. All the time. Human errors. But lies about cancer

are always positive lies; kind lies. 'The treatment has been most successful.'
Robin was a surgically-revealed cancer case.

The discarded flowers, heads askance, drooped over the top of the black sack. The goldfish whirled giddily round in the freshly aereated water.

'If it's not cancer, then what is it? Please! What is it?'

Don't sound desperate. She may be panicked into silence. I waited, stunned by anticipation of further shock.

It came. Subtle as a caber from a catapult.

'Maggots!' she said firmly.

My heart syncopated. Somersaulted. Steadied.

'Maggots?' I found I was repeating myself. 'Maggots? What on earth have maggots got to do with it? What maggots?'

'Mr Kissane, our Pathologist. He showed a jar to Sr Ryan today. It contained maggots. They were cultured from a swab taken from Robin's surgical wound. It seems,' she limped on weakly, 'it seems, that perhaps he swallowed a fly.'

He-swallowed-a-fly; do-you-think-he'll-die, poor-Robin-Heron. I choked.

'But – a fly? It would be destroyed by gastric juices, surely? I mean, a fly wouldn't mean . . .' I gagged on the word, '. . . it wouldn't mean – maggots?'

'It must have been a bluebottle. And somehow the eggs developed in the intestines and became active when Robin was exposed to surgery.'

Sweet Jesus, no! Heavy crawling slow-moving maggots. Repulsive white bloated bodies, tiny brown heads. Bloated bodies, gorging blood and flesh. Robin's flesh! Jesus, no!

I felt myself go very cold. Blue-ice cold.

Tiny goose pimples prickled my face; my bare arms.

Follicles of hair rose all over my head and body. Rigid pinnacles of petrified skin.

I smelled my own fear.

I leaned my rigid body against the sink.

Nurse Gilligan sounded far away. Her voice a confliction of concern and apprehension. Through an audial haze, I heard her speak. 'You're all right, Mrs Heron, aren't you? Do you feel okay? I mean, you won't let on I mentioned it to you?'

I dragged myself out of purdah and touched her arm in reassurance. 'It's strictly off the record. I won't say a word.' My voice quavered.

The door swung closed behind her.

Internal rotting. Putrefying flesh, eaten away. This is primeval. Heinous horror. Nauseating. Revolting. Living crawling tissue . . .

The spastic trance splintered and shattered.

I retched. Holding the taps of the sluice, I gripped on, as my stomach vomited up its protest. Disgorged half-digested food. Purged itself of everything until only bile splattered the white earthenware.

In a reflex somnambulance, I swished it away and cleaned the sink bowl.

Bankruptcy of courage.

Fear of facing Robin. Fear of revulsion. Recoil.

Could one feel revulsion for the victim? I didn't know. Revulsion for the writhing mass that might be swarming beneath the gamgee pad? I didn't know.

There is no fear but fear of fear itself. Good old Inez! Soldier on! Step it out, girl! Trample it underfoot! Jesus, where are you now? Bob! Nathan! Help me! Someone, help, help!

Slowly I walked to No 10.

Deliberately I steeled myself to look at Robin, fearful of my reaction.

He was asleep.

I felt a swamping upsurge of love.

My shaking hands sloshed the water tank on to the shelf. Bob lifted it. 'I think we can go now,' he said softly. 'He seems peaceful.'

'I've something to tell you. Something quite horrible. You'll have to brace yourself for it.'

'Do you want me to stop the car?' Bob glanced in the driving mirror.

'Yes. Yes, please.' He pulled in to the kerb. The engine cut to silence. In the darkness beneath the trees, my words teetered out like summer-sprayed midges splotched on a windscreen.

When I had finished, Bob spoke. 'But it just can't be true. I mean, how could these things have lived that length of time? All right, I know nothing of the medical aspects, but looking at it logically – how *could* it happen?'

His voice revealed nothing of his feelings. His skin was ochre-tinged.

Suddenly my body flamed with candescent heat. The dry retching started again. Bob scrambled out and helped me from the passenger seat.

When my stomach settled, we clung together – linked in a nexus of horror.

'Bob. We must never mention this again. Never. It's enough to drive one to insanity. From now on, I'm not going to think of it. I'm putting this hour behind me forever. I'm going to live life fully, come what may. But this hour is behind us. Agreed?'

He nodded emphatically. Then propounded a theory. 'There's just one thing that might make sense of it,' he said slowly, pockmarking his words with pauses. 'Jeff McMahon did refer to a "bug". Maybe this,' he gulped, 'this maggot creature or whatever it is, maybe it's a natural development of the "bug".'

SEVEN

July, August, September

'His withered fist still knocking
at Death's door.'

Thomas Sackville, Earl of Dorset
(*Mirour for Magistrates*)

A montage of pictures, audio-visual, invaded my sleep . . .

. . . Voices from the house next door. Neighbours calling goodbyes to friends.

'There's a wasps' nest under the aubrietia. Tomorrow, we'll burn them out.'

Immolation. A holocaust of live torches rising from flaming blue flowers . . .

. . . Black linoleum on the kitchen floor, patterned in a galaxy of floral sprays. Cleaning; vacuum-suctioned air. Underneath, I unearthed a clutch of maggots feeding in the damp on a lost rasher-rind . . .

. . . Religious Knowledge class. Herod consumed by maggots devouring his living flesh. Titus, destroyer of the Temple, destroyed by a mite boring into his brain. 'Vengeance is mine', saith the Lord, 'I will repay.' . . .

. . . Sausages sizzling in a pan; the grocer had been careless. Grilled grubs wriggled frantically from under the sheathing skin . . .

. . . West Africa. *Dracunculus medinensis.* Parasitic infestation from contaminated drinking water. Migration from the intestine. A slender worm. She settles under the skin near the ankle. Medical cure: phenothiazine. Local cure: 'Stand in water. She'll come out to lay her eggs. Then wind a stick around her body. It will take at least a week to lure her out completely.' . . .

. . . I dipped my fork into the spaghetti, flavoured with tomato sauce. Raised it to my mouth. A movement caught my eye. Hypnotised, I looked. A heaving organic mass of squelched maggots. A whirling carousel of white bodies garnished in blood. Bisected granules of pus; writhing in rhythm . . .

. . . Goldfish. Bloated with fungus. Cavorting crazily in a tank of hot water. A gas jet fired the temperature up up – hotter, hotter . . .

I woke. My body was burning. My skin steamed beneath a film of sweat. The night was over.

'Inez! Inez, are you all right?' Bob took me in his arms and held me, stroking my hair, comforting me like a child, until the horror receded.

In the afternoon, a stranger came to see Robin. An elderly well-groomed man with thinning silver hair brushed back from his forehead. Smooth and plausible, courteous yet decisive in manner. Professor O'Grady, Consultant Physician.

I waited. 'I'm just going to have a word with Dr Monaghan,' he said.

A half-hour passed. I saw them stroll to the car park. Dr Monaghan carried a manila file. His head was bent towards the professor, listening – hand gesticulating occasionally in silent mime. A final wave and the professor drove away.

Dr Monaghan called me to the Nurses' Station. I sat down and he closed the door.

'Better brains than mine have been intensively active on Robin's case in the past few days. They suggest something like this. Last year, Robin may have swallowed a bluebottle. It lodged in the intestines and disgorged its eggs. These foreign bodies naturally set up action in the tissue; tumours. Surgery removed these tumours. But the grubs damaged the intestines and continue to do so.'

I blessed Nurse Gilligan for her advance warning. Future shock was now past shock. If the tumours were not malignant, then rationally the future, if there were to be a future, would be brighter?

Dr Monaghan was still speaking. 'By lucky chance, I was able to contact Professor O'Grady. When I was a student, he did a year's research on a drug which acts on the chemical substance which this type of grub produces. We plan to use this drug, and also one we have here at Bramble Grange for leukaemia. Now, Mrs Heron, I emphasise that this is the way it *appears* to be. We haven't ruled out other causes. An intestinal amoeba, for instance. But we're looking into that.'

Harnessed hope was released and surged over my face. He recognised it. The thin kind features grew troubled.

'I *must* emphasise that Robin is very very low. An extremely sick child. But there is one good thing. These grubs cannot reproduce themselves. They appear to be located in the abdomen only. The question is, at this very late hour, can they be killed off by drugs and the damage repaired before Robin's resistance collapses?'

With nightfall, my terror returned. I telephoned Nathan.

'They've mentioned an amoeba, though they think it's unlikely. Could you educate me?'

He sounded startled. 'Well, an amoeba is a tiny creature. A protozoan, little more than twenty-five microns – that's 1/1000th inch in diameter. It's ingested in raw food or contaminated water and it can break through the lining of the intestines.'

'Can it reproduce itself, Nathan?'

'It hasn't a conventional sex life, as such. It's a single cell animal, like a blob of jelly – a semi-fluid substance with a nucleus. It reproduces by dividing into halves which then mature into adult amoebae.'

'They're working on that theory. But they think it's unlikely to be the cause of Robin's troubles.'

'Very unlikely,' he agreed. 'The symptoms vary greatly in different patients. But, while it's common in the tropics and subtropics, it's a very very rare condition in this country.'

Stumbling over the words, I briefed him on the bluebottle and grubs situation.

'This is quite extraordinary, Inez. Normally these foreign bodies are utterly destroyed by gastric juices.' He paused. 'You know, you are very fortunate in the team Robin has. Professor O'Grady is a highly respected man; rightly so. Jeff McMahon is expending himself far in excess of what could be expected of him. He is literally trying absolutely everything and following all the trails. As to Dr Monaghan, he's remarkably honest to have told you all this so frankly. He must have recognised your calibre and stoicism.'

'Nathan, I'm not stoical. I'm terrified. I'm afraid even to go to bed. Afraid of dreams that could drive me to insanity. These grubs – maggots – they've opened a whole new spectrum of subconscious horror . . .'

He cut in before I could elaborate. 'I know. Now listen to me. What you must do, Inez, is to expunge this maggot business from your mind. It sounds revolting, yes. But, in fact, in World War One, maggots were used to combat and heal chronic septic wounds.'

'A symbiotic relationship? On the principle of the witch doctors?'

'Basically, yes. But, Inez, it's very minor. Of no importance to the outcome. Gruesome to dwell on but of little significance.'

He switched direction. 'Do you have a transistor radio?'

The change of subject surprised me. 'Why yes, but . . .'

'Good. Now tune in to something soothing when you've taken your sleeping pill. Music. Just let your mind go blank. Let the music roll over you. Drift with it. You will try that, won't you?'

Tchaikovsky's Symphony No. 6. 'The Pathetique' 1st Movement.

It worked. Dreamless sleep.

For two weeks, Robin held his tenuous grip on life. Drips were shifted as the veins collapsed. Nathan wasn't too disturbed by this. 'It's not always easy to find a vein in a child. But it's almost always possible,' he said.

I.V. feeding from various bottles. *Sterivac* – a clear fluid. *Intralipid* 10% – a cloudy chalk white substance. *Aminosol Glucose* – dark yellow.

Dr Hunter took more blood samples. 'Robin's doing nicely. The immediate problem is nutritional. We'll have to maintain the present level. But this,' he held up the phial of blood, 'this will give a clearer picture. The internal damage, though, is pretty extensive.'

Stitches in the feet; the groin.

The abdominal wound healed. The sutures were removed.

Dr Monaghan's vulpine face was open, candid. 'Robin seems to be holding his own. We're certain a housefly was involved, as I mentioned to you. But it may have been secondary. Certainly some parasite initially caused the trouble.'

'But you inherited Robin's case as a lymphosarcoma. The diagnosis was given. The definition was malignant tumours.'

'Well, it's a parasite,' he reiterated. 'The exact breakdown isn't identified. Whatever it is, it responded to radium. The surgery in June this year was to rectify a fairly routine post-operative condition – a problem with the gut. This, unfortunately, often happens and the intestines stick to the abdominal wall. But, if Robin makes it, the long-term future is infinitely brighter now. Admittedly, his temperature goes up and down a bit. But it's never very high. The peak is about 101.'

I brushed back my tears with my hand. 'Thank you for giving me the low-down in layman's language.'

He shied away from my emotionalism. 'There is no other language.'

'There is, you know, Dr Monaghan. There's the cryptic answer. The evasive reply that tells the half-truth.'

Some days were fairly good. Some less so. It was necessary to cut down on the sedatives. The pain increased in strength.

Jeff McMahon explained. 'I'm anxious that Robin should pass water, and start to eat and drink. The antibiotics can be fed intravenously through the drip. That should relieve his discomfort a little.'

The hawthorn blossoms turned from creamy ivory to brown. Mid-July tinctures of autumn. Dark-winged sycamore seeds grew in thick clusters, soon to be released in flight that would bring new life beneath the winter's earth.

An injection was given to help urination. The drip speed was increased. Robin's arms and hands began to tremble. He vomited four times in as many hours. The bowl was removed for the contents to be measured.

He lay, staring at his fingers. He scratched patterns on the raw pink skin of his life-line.

Captured. Confused. Pain . . .

En route home, I passed two small boys, jam-jars clutched in hot sticky hands. Inside, honey bees buzzed deliriously. Blurred brown and yellow bodies, trapped as they had drifted through the waving fronds of powdered pollen. Glass cages with tiny sieved ventilation holes in the metal lids. The delicate beauty of fucshia blooms, scarlet petals and purple stilletoes, carpeted on wilting green leaves.

I stopped the car. Coins changed hands. The bees staggered out unsurely. They spread their wings in whirring flight and soared away to freedom.

Blood money buying life.

Everything has its price . . .

'You're so friendly and approachable. You're going to have a problem when you're a big-brass senior consultant,' I stopped Dr Hunter on the passage.

The cherubic face broke into a ready smile. 'That's a while off, as yet. Look, go down to the sitting-room. I've one patient to see and then I'll be with you.'

He came in, taking a menthol cigarette from a packet. He lit it; then sat down and leaned back in the chair.

'Robin should be all right for the night. I've ordered an injection that will ensure a good sleep.'

'He's had a bad day.'

'I know. Because of yesterday's pain, we had to slow down the drip. Now it's in arrears and we've accelerated it to catch up on his intake,' he explained.

'What's the picture?' I prompted.

He drew a bulky wad of pharmaceutical pamphlets from his bulging pocket. 'Well, I know more about nutrition than I ever expected to. Robin's receiving three thousand calories a day – enough to keep a strong man ploughing a field.' He inhaled, then relaxed. 'He's been unsettled for the last few days. That's why we've been easing up on the drugs and antibiotics in the hope his own antibodies will start doing the job for themselves.'

'And how's it going?'

'Indications are that his healing powers are getting to work. The drain is drying, and so is the abdominal wound – as you'll have seen. An abscess *has* formed but we can treat that. You know, in another person, the present situation would be critical. But with Robin's extraordinary restorative powers, there is – in the light of present circumstances and bearing in mind all that's happened to him – well, there's definite hope, I feel.'

'I see. What about the vomiting?'

'It may be due to the drugs. That's part of the reason for reducing them.' He fiddled with the cigarette packet. 'Now, as to the parasite. It hasn't been fully identified. Normally one would assume that the gastric juices would have destroyed it in transit through the stomach. The drugs which we've used haven't flushed them all out yet. We're still finding them in his faeces. Definitely there are still some there. Surgery revealed little tumours; tiny things which appear to have burrowed into the gut. They've lain dormant. The mystery is how they've managed to survive so long.'

He continued thoughtfully. 'Now, take the example of a fly . . .'

'An ordinary housefly? *Musca domestica?*'

'Exactly. Egg to larva to grub to housefly. Yet all these parasites we've been finding are at one stage in their metamorphosis. Their development is to one point, though they differ in size. It's unequivocally established that they cannot reproduce themselves.'

'Like amoebae, they've no sex life?'

He grinned through an exhalation of smoke. 'Absolutely nil. But the rest is quite honestly out of my field and into a vet's.'

He gathered up his scattered papers. 'After second surgery here at Bramble Grange – that was Robin's fifth operation, wasn't it . . . ?'

I nodded.

'Well,' he went on, 'Mr McMahon recognised that it was a parasite. The picture was very black. Pretty well hopeless. But it seems a bit brighter now. Professor O'Grady is working on a serum for the parasite. And we plan tomorrow that Robin should have some physiotherapy. We want to get his legs moving again.'

'The drip seems to have affected them adversely,' I agreed.

He looked up appraisingly. His eyes assessed me. 'You've a remarkably clear understanding of the situation.'

I passed the compliment back to his camp. 'That's because you all keep us up to date on each problem as it arises. Our daughter, Helen, is brain-damaged. We've learned to face life's realities. People speak of "acceptance". It's an anomaly. There is no rejection of the truth, the reality. One must accept it; but it's easier to confront it when one knows what's happening.'

A white-coated woman came next day. Her manner was professionally brusque. 'I'm the physiotherapist.'

'Shall I leave you?'

'If you would, please.'

Robin's eyes were dark pools of terror. He started to moan. Then broke into sobs.

Her tone mellowed a little. 'Robin, it's just a couple of movements for your legs. Your mother can practise them with you after I've gone.'

Later she explained. 'Try to get him to wriggle his toes. He keeps his limbs so rigid. We have to get them exercising again.'

She left, saying, 'I'll be back tomorrow. Same time.'

By 'tomorrow', his condition had deteriorated. There was no question of physiotherapy.

An air-filled mattress was installed. It was electrically controlled and purred like a softly revving engine. The panel had red lights, weight control, and a dial knob tuned to 'heavy'.

Dr Monaghan showed concern. 'Robin's temperature is running high and his pulse is fast. I don't feel we can keep him going indefinitely on that drip. It would appear there's a blockage somewhere; that may be why he's vomiting quite a lot. Added to that, he's very dehydrated, at the moment.'

'Where do you begin to tackle all these problems, doctor?'

'It's a question of trying to balance the I.V. feeding. From recent blood tests, we've worked out a formula which should work in the drip. But the parasite is there. Dormant, but not dismissed.'

Robin was settling into sleep when a very old priest appeared in the doorway of No 10.

'I'm a Jesuit Father, from Gardiner Street. I'd like to bless Robin with this crucifix. It belonged to Fr John Sullivan – a miracle worker if ever there was one.'

Robin's head swivelled round at the whispered sounds. The eyes dilated with the familiar fear of intruders. 'Get out! Get out, I say!' he shrieked.

Flushing with embarrassment, Bob stood up and moved out to the passage. 'Robin gets very upset with strangers,' he explained. 'I'm sorry.'

The childish voice shrilled demandingly. 'Daddy! Dad! I want you here. Come back. Right now.' The treble cracked into a whimpering.

I sat immobile, a synthetic smile frozen round my mouth. I felt a primitive urge to scratch and tear the skin of my face. I forced myself to grip the bedrail.

The soutaned figure reappeared with Bob. 'I'll remember you, Robin, in my Masses and prayers,' he said softly. He turned to me.

'Sure I remember them all. I visit all the hospitals, you know. Go round with the crucifix blessing all the sick. Just put this relic under the child's pillow and I'll pray for him.'

The old grey head nodded as he pleaded. 'Maybe another time you'll let me bless you, Robin?'

My voice, croaking with fury, murmured social thanks.

I felt hate. A positive physical condition. The maelstrom swirled, blinding me. Then ebbed.

I was drained.

The evening sky was a vivid pink. It caught and reflected the irridescent varnish on my nails. *The darkest hours. Overcome these and you can conquer anything.*

The Samaritans' brief to desperate callers: 'Try to hang on for another sixty seconds.'

Robin had flopped over. He was dozing on his pillows.

I half-hoped he was dead.

The trunk of Robin's body began to swell. The sunken ribs vanished. The legs, limp on the sheets, were withered rickety twigs.

Each night, Nurse Gilligan massaged his heels tenderly and rested the knobbly ankles on rings of cotton wool.

Dr Hunter looked in. Outside a steady drizzle was falling. He touched my arm. 'Come out a moment. I want to talk to you.'

'Do I imagine it or is Robin's tummy distended?'

'You're right. He's a bit liverish and jaundiced, I'm afraid. I'm not sure of the cause. There may be several. It's not surprising, I suppose, since we're feeding so much intravenously. But it's not good. I have to warn you. I feel, well – I feel he's slipping back.'

Within days the skin had yellowed. His body trembled frequently, convulsively. He vomited more frequently.

Dr Hunter tried to analyse it. 'The trembling may be a result of withdrawal from opiates. We had to try it when he seemed to be improving. We had to give him a chance.'

'Are things critical now?'

He rubbed his chin. 'I don't think the danger of death is imminent. But I'm no prophet.'

A Ryle's tube was reinserted down Robin's nose to the stomach.

'At least he'll have the comfort of drinking without vomiting,' Sr Ryan said. Her voice was sad.

A portable X-ray unit was wheeled in.

Robin's shaking hand reached out for water. Thin yellow blisters had formed on his lips. He slurped the glass. 'Try to lift me up please, Mum. I'm terrified of this trembling.'

That evening the X-ray plates were clipped to the viewing box in the Nurses' Station. One, a centre-cut of the trunk, diminuitive; a child's frame, photographed from navel to waist. Another, upwards from the waist. Only the vertebrae of the spine and the rib-cage were decipherable. A dark shadow curved in a half-arc up towards the ribs, long and thick. The exacerbated liver? I didn't know.

The body on the bed was very blown up now. All the veins showed; blue ribbons of life, pellucid through yellowed skin. The wound, a pale purple splash on saffron tissue.

Robin's breathing was fast and shallow. Panting.

The jaundice became more manifest daily. His voice thickened with phlegm. His eyes clouded in a murky pellicle. Mucous-lined mouth blew bubbles of spittled froth as the weak voice broke through. His voice had the cracked timbre of the very old.

'I'm going to cough.'

'There now. You're all right.'

'I'm not all right. I'm past it. I'm dying.' He wheezed gently. 'Dear Heaven. I'm dead.'

Scrawny clawlike fingers dragged at the steel bedframe above his head. 'My toes feel terrible. I'm afraid of falling back.'

The pillows, four of them now, propped him up. Yet his body kept slipping down again. A bolster was wedged below his feet.

Sr Ryan reviewed the position one morning. Robin's bed had been wheeled away for further diagnostic X-rays of his body.

'He had four ounces of tea this morning. We aspirated him beforehand but not afterwards. It stayed down. You know, Mrs Heron, he's almost unique. His body fights so hard that, as long as there's life, I feel there's hope. Genuinely so. He's virtually indestructible.'

'Nathan, what's happening?' I had narrated the liver deterioration to him.

'There are tubes which carry bile from the stomach via the liver to the upper part of the intestine,' he explained. 'These appear to be becoming blocked. The bile might be seeping from the liver into the body and so causing the abdominal swelling. The trembling is due to toxic poisoning.'

'Bad, isn't it?'

'Well, I had a patient once who lasted six weeks with a jaundiced liver. But it's pretty nearly hopeless. The drip is probably a saline solution to avoid dehydration. You understand that problem, don't you, Inez?'

'I do. I seem to understand everything – and nothing. I know now that much of this suffering need never have happened to Robin. Just human error; misdiagnosis.'

'You don't sound bitter . . .'

'I don't feel bitterness, Nathan. Just regret and a terrible bleak sadness. Litigation, financial compensation – they've flashed through my mind. But it's all so pointless. Money is God. But, like God, it cannot buy back the past.'

Surgeon, physician, radiotherapist: all had differing views. All were honest enough to express them.

Jeff McMahon was characteristically succinct. 'I feel the demerits of the parasitic treatment may be exceeding its advantages. Last-ditch surgery could be necessary if the quantity of bile accumulation from the new blockage doesn't diminish in the next forty-eight hours.'

He read the aversion to surgery in my face. 'It won't be as severe as the fistulas job,' he continued. 'That was the second operation I did – Robin's fifth. I think the jaundiced condition of the liver may be partially due to this drug. It appears to be effective in controlling, though not removing, this parasite.'

Professor O'Grady felt Robin's abdomen. He listened with his stethoscope. 'There appears to be less fluid there.'

Dr Monaghan was non-commital. 'Robin's spirits seem a little improved. He was reading this morning.' He hesitated. 'We've ordered another blood transfusion. It will start tonight.'

A suppository. Robin's bowels moved promptly, a glutinous yellow substance on the sheets. A nurse scraped up the faecal mess with a spatula and put it into a carton for laboratory analysis.

Two more blood transfusions.

Blue lobellia, white alyssum and scarlet salvia blazed in a plethora of colour outside. Crimson roses shed darkening petals on the smooth green lawn.

My spirits were dead as the spent flowers.

The forty-eight hours passed. Jeff McMahon made no further reference to surgery. A week went by; it was August now.

Dr Monaghan called me to the sitting room. 'It's a while since I've seen you, Mrs Heron. I haven't been avoiding you but I've been getting in touch with a lot of people about Robin . . .'

'You're a busy man and you've many other patients,' I interrupted him. It sounded obsequious. I meant it sincerely.

'Anyway, I want to talk to you now,' he said.

I stood by the window. Waiting.

'As I see it, the blockage isn't complete. The jaundice is controlled although it fluctuates in intensity, even in twelve hours.' He paused, in his own deliberate way. 'As to the parasite. It hasn't yet been identified. But it's being analysed at the Nevers Hospital in Dundalk where they deal with tropical diseases.' He glanced across at me. 'You know there's a question of surgery?'

'Yes! And I know what I feel about it. Veto!' I said vehemently.

He nodded. 'It seems to me that the trouble from the parasite only follows surgery – as though exposure to air activates these mites that otherwise lie dormant. When surgery was involved back in June, all the complications of the parasite followed. I feel that radiotherapy was successful before, when Robin first came to Bramble Grange last year. Now he *has* had rather a lot of radium, but a small amount might prove useful in killing off the remaining mites.'

The spectre of surgery seemed to creep over me. Evening shadows fell across the parklands, touching the trees and lawns. The sky was a silver pearl-grey. I felt chilled though the room was warmed by the residual heat of the day.

I sat down slowly. 'God! Not surgery again. Please try anything. But not surgery.'

Dr Monaghan went on. 'I feel that surgery means sinuses, infections, abscesses, etcetera. It seems to me that Robin doesn't respond too well to it. And I think that indications are, from the clearing up of wounds and external healing, that Robin may be healing inside. Naturally, as a surgeon, Mr McMahon thinks in terms of operating . . .'

'As a physician thinks in terms of treatment? And you, as a radio-therapist, turn to radium. Well, as a layman – and Robin's mother – I can only see that if he's going to die, it's better that he slips away naturally rather than experience all the pain and suffering that are synonymous with surgery. Particularly if it's of doubtful advant-age.'

There was silence. I looked up at him. The sharply etched face was grieved. 'You know, Mrs Heron, there may reach a stage when we just have to recognise and accept the Will of God.'

From anyone else, I would have recoiled at the negativity. From him, it touched me. I realised the depth of respect and affection I had for this gentle man.

'Look, Dr Monaghan, if you're away at a clinic, could you leave word at the Station to contact us before considering surgery. You could say we'd prefer to defer it for the time being at least.'

'I'll do that, of course. Don't worry. Nothing would be done without consulting you.'

Bob felt differently. Less subjective and emotional than I did. 'I think we should keep an open mind. Be guided by the experts.'

'But when they differ?'

'The next few days may decide it for us. We'll see then.'

Robin's face puffed out. He was on steroids.

Dr Monaghan allowed himself a little cautious optimism. 'I'm reasonably satisfied that the cortisone is breaking down the obstruction. The aspiration of bile from the stomach is diminishing, and the last swab culture was negative. We'll keep radiotherapy in reserve, as it's rather severe.'

Pain grew in intensity. Nothing could alleviate it. Three injections in an hour but it continued unabated.

Sr Ryan came and sat beside Robin. He turned his bloated tear-drenched face to her and clutched her dress. 'Sister, please. You've got to do something!'

The strong hand quietly stroked his forehead. 'Robin, if I give you any more, I'll kill you.'

He pulled his head away. 'Go on, then. Kill me. I want to die anyway.'

A bitter-sweet smile flickered across her face. 'After all the work we've put into getting you better? We couldn't do that, could we?'

She returned with a filled syringe, and spoke to me pianissimo. 'This is the most I can do.'

Injection. She sat with his hand in hers until he fell asleep.

A few days later, Dr Hunter breezed in. 'Come on. Down to the sitting-room again, Mrs Heron!'

I followed him. 'I've had various blood tests taken,' he began. 'Tomorrow there'll be more. There *is* an increase in pain. The parasitic obstruction is near the duodenum and is backing up the bile in the stomach which can't function properly. Mr McMahon feels surgery is essential. It will clear the jaundiced condition of the liver. Radiotherapy would do extensive damage, he considers.'

I was about to reiterate my views but he stalled me. 'Now listen. A look around – a little look around – will reveal the condition of the peritoneum and other general situations about which we can otherwise only guess. Professor O'Grady agrees, because with steroids we can only do so much and no more. There is an abscess but we hope to treat it with antibiotics to which it should respond. But that would be after surgery,' he added.

'So surgery it has to be?' I had lived on the periphery of hope. Now again it was eroding. Black fear and despair broke in a wave.

'Cigarette?' He opened a packet and passed it to me, playing for time. It was empty. 'It's my cadging trick!' he spoofed.

I gave a nervous laugh. 'Have one of mine.' I rooted in my handbag. 'You know, you're a psychologist as well as a surgeon.'

'Well, it's good to hear you laugh.' He flicked his lighter into flame. 'Mrs Heron, Robin can't go on in this condition,' he said more seriously. 'We're having problems with the drip again. Now, Robin's healing powers are quite spectacular. They appear to be sufficient at the moment to respond after surgery.'

I was silent.

He said speculatively. 'You know, it might have been better if we'd gone ahead and operated two weeks ago.'

There was no reply to that.

A shadow at the door of No 10. A white-coated man in a brilliantly flowered shirt. Lank and lean, with a full pouting mouth and eyes hazed behind tinted glasses.

Sr Ryan introduced us. 'This is our Pathologist, Mr Kissane. Cecil – Mrs Heron.'

He took my hand in his long bony fingers. 'I've rather an odd question for you, Mrs Heron. It's related to your Christian name. Inez, isn't it? Spanish?'

'Yes. Iberian, you could say. Portuguese or Spanish, depending on the spelling. Agnes in English! Una in Irish. But I'm native Gael for over a century back.'

'You've no Spanish connections? No contact with Spanish possessions or tropical countries?' he persisted.

'None at all. The furthest I've ever been was Israel. And that's ten years ago. A last splurge before I was married – or pregnant!'

'I see,' he smiled. 'It was just an off-chance. I thought it might give us a lead. You see, we've had Robin's tissues from Holy Innocents'. We've sent specimens to Stormont Veterinary Research. To Liverpool and London. Other spots too. Loosely speaking, the larvae produced are of the fly type. That's the culture from the swabs, I mean.'

'Which leaves you a choice of one of eighty-five thousand species ranging from the Arctic tundra to the Sahara sands?' I had researched a radio feature once, on the subject of flies.

'Dead right. They could be indigenous to these islands but possibly they are tropical. From a pathological viewpoint, I feel that if the medical men can retain life long enough, undoubtedly we'll be able to act and effectively remove these parasites. The problem, clinically, is Robin's poor condition.'

His speech was languid, casually lazy. Instinctively I responded to his easy manner. 'So for you, Mr Kissane, it's a question of identification?'

'Just that. Usually it's a case of flushing out with the appropriate drug. Children frequently swallow things – worms or other infestations of one or another sort. You see, there's a breakdown of parasites into world classes. In Egypt, or Saudi-Arabia, you might find one type of fluke. In South America, another kind. You haven't been to the United States?' he added, hopefully.

'No. Never.'

'Mmmm.' He sucked in his lower lip. 'It was just a thought. There is a parasitic fly there – the screw fly – in the Mississippi region.'

'Robin had never been out of Ireland when this whole trouble started last year.'

He had opened channels to a whole new vista. Anxiously I tried to lay paving stones to further communication. 'You will tell me of developments, won't you, Mr Kissane?'

'Sure! My Pathology Lab is just beyond the Nurses' Station. You pass it every time you come down Ward P.'

'I thought Pathology was located downstairs. Near Out-patients.'

'It's blood you're thinking of. They look after that down below. My speciality is specimens. Urine, faeces, and all that,' he smiled wryly.

'And swab cultures?' I ventured. 'They're yours too?'

'That's right.'

This then must be the man. The man who had first stumbled on the maggot development. This gangling specialist with the easy camaradie and sensuous mouth.

'So the bluebottle? The grubs . . . ?' I couldn't finish the words.

'Yes. Perhaps, in a way, that was fortuitous. A housefly *did* lay its eggs. Usually they do in mid-summer. About a hundred, it's estimated. It must have settled on the wound – you know the way Robin tends to lie sometimes with his pyjamas open. It was possibly about July. A freak chance – but it happened! We then got on the right track, I think. A parasitic infestation of some sort. An insect. Or maybe a nematode, a worm of some kind. Now it's a case of finding positive identification.'

I felt it could not be in better hands.

The divergence of views became more apparent. Feelings were taking entrenched positions.

Bob had an open mind. I couldn't see beyond the pain and suffering of surgery. Dr Monaghan and Jeff McMahon also viewed the situation differently.

Dr Monaghan talked to me. 'Personally I feel that surgery merely to by-pass an obstruction is insufficient reason for such a major act. Robin's deterioration has been less marked this last week. And radiotherapy worked before!'

'Well, how about compromise? Radiotherapy now, with the possibility of surgery in the future – if it becomes essential?'

'I don't much like the idea.' He offered no elaboration.

I shrugged helplessly. 'We've no one to guide us. Our G.P. hasn't been in contact since Robin first became ill.' I gambled, dicing on his strength and kindness. 'Dr Monaghan, it's like this. Robin came here as your patient. You gave him a remission. Now you've brought us within sight of hope for recovery. Will you regard him as your patient, or is that unorthodox for you?'

An unpretentious wave of the hand. The thin face showed the conflict of his humanity with the crisis which was looming.

'You know, Mrs Heron, there's another danger. Being realistic, this drip could cause a clot which might knock Robin out any time. Today, tomorrow, any moment. It's a critical situation. And they wouldn't be removing the blockage; merely by-passing it.'

'So?'

'Well – I'll think about it.'

I felt relief.

Bob was uncertain. He telephoned Jeff McMahon.

'A second opinion is quite welcome, as far as I'm concerned,' the consultant said cogently.

'We're sorry this divergence of views has arisen over Robin. We've the highest regard for both yourself and Dr Monaghan . . .'

'And I have the greatest respect for Dr Monaghan in his own field,' Mr McMahon interjected. 'But radiotherapy is for the treatment of malignancies and this is *not* a malignancy.'

'If Robin were your child, what would you do?' Bob ventured.

'I'd call another opinion.'

'And who finds "another opinion"?'

'You do.' Mr McMahon was direct. 'You do, through your G.P.'

Bob was silent for a moment. The surgeon continued. 'The position is grave. The drip is inserted in a deep vein. When, or if, it packs up, we're in serious trouble. Now I'm not suggesting that surgery is the answer to everything,' he qualified, 'but, in my view, it's the only answer at the moment.'

Bob was converted.

Parental impasse.

Professional impasse.

I phoned Nathan from Bramble Grange. 'Come and see me on your way home. We can discuss it then,' he quietly reassured me.

Dr Hunter was bowling along the passage as we left. 'It's been a day of phone calls,' he said, 'but we all seem agreed that an independent decision is best.'

'We'll certainly abide by it,' Bob replied.

'Time is of importance now,' Dr Hunter emphasised.

Nathan was sitting by the fire in his sanctum. The clutter of books and paintings were comforting. A supper tray was ready.

I told him of developments.

'By-passing the duodenum means taking up a piece of the small intestine and attaching it to the stomach. You detour round the obstruction,' he explained. 'Now the problem with the vein is that when you've used the highest part of the limb – in Robin's case, at the groin – you can't use the lower leg for a time. It would reject it.'

'That's why he sometimes feels soreness in the leg and pain in his toes?'

'Exactly. The vein is protesting. It's dangerous because the vein could give up or there could be an embolus – that is, a clot. Such a situation *must* be rectified. Indefinite dependence on I.V. feeding is impossible. Robin must be given his chance to take nutrition orally. And that means surgery.'

'Can you make any suggestions re another opinion?' I asked. The mystery of Nathan's past life obviously excluded him from filling that role.

His reply came promptly. 'When I had surgery some years ago, Norman Kelso of the Alexandra Hospital operated. I would have complete faith in his judgment. Added to that, he's a Trinity College Graduate. Not National University, as are the others.'

'None of the Alumni loyalties would arise? The old-boy network, you mean?'

'That's it.'

'So what should we do next, Nathan?'

'I think you should inform both Dr Monaghan and Mr McMahon of your wishes. They'll invite Mr Kelso in to view Robin's case. And, you know, there's a relief to both of them in having the decision taken out of their hands.'

That night I wrote two letters. One to Dr Monaghan; the other to Jeff McMahon. Early next morning, I left them at Bramble Grange reception desk. Addressed and marked 'Urgent – re Robin Heron'.

They were duplicate notes, explaining our divergent views, as parents; and suggesting that Mr Kelso be invited to give his opinion.

Late that afternoon, Mr Kelso came to examine Robin. I waited in the Preparation room opposite the Station. Dr Monaghan was away at an out-of-town clinic.

I could see Jeff McMahon in conversation with a small military-moustached man. Dr Hunter leafed through a file. The Station door was closed.

Presently Dr Hunter called me in and made introductions. Then he left.

Jeff McMahon stood silently, leaning against the desk; a one-man audience of hypnotic eyes watching the on-stage players.

Mr Kelso wasted no words. 'From the files, it is a case quite beyond my experience. I can only give my views in relation to what I've seen and read.' His thin girlish hands tapped the desk. 'It's quite remarkable that the I.V. drip has been maintained for such a length of time . . .'

'It's a tribute to Mr McMahon,' I interjected.

The tawny amber eyes held mine briefly in acknowledgment.

Mr Kelso continued. 'The vein is very ominous. The only alterna-tive vein, now, is in the neck. A very messy undesirable business.'

The crunch was coming. I braced myself.

He continued. 'Robin is an extremely sick child – a critically ill child. In my view, surgery is absolutely essential to effect a by-pass of the blockage. Nutriment must start orally and the sooner the better. Surgery is the only way to achieve this.'

It was Nathan's verdict, uttered almost verbatim.

'And radiotherapy?' I was being won over, but in Dr Monaghan's absence I had to make the point.

'Radiotherapy has the disadvantage of doing much damage before it could begin to break down the blockage. And there's another warning to be born in mind. The seepage which is coming through the rectum from the bowels, is only seepage. Just that. There's no way of judging the condition of the lower part of the intestine. Surgery would show that.'

'I understand. So your opinion is . . . ?'

'My final word is that surgery is essential. And promptly,' he added.

Dr Hunter clarified the details that night.

'Mr McMahon has surgery at St Victor's all day tomorrow. The only available time would be 7.30 p.m. It's inadvisable so late in the evening. So he intends to operate on Robin on Saturday morning.'

One day to D Day.

Saturday: a deluge of rain. A few intrepid housewives held their umbrellas knee-high to escape the mechanised ablution. A besodden policeman pedalled his bicycle through a swell of high-flying spray.

I swung into Bramble Grange. Jeff McMahon's car was parked under the dripping trees.

Ward P was Saturday-quiet. Sr Ryan came out of the Station.

'Robin was quite cheerful going off. Of course, he didn't have a very clear mind. We'd given him a pre-med this morning. I went with him to Theatre. He gave me a wink and said, "This will probably do some good now and I'll be able to eat again." He was almost asleep when I left him.'

I wandered down to the sitting-room. Robin's door was partially open. His trolley and chattels were evicted on to the passage. I heard the swish of deck brushes; the slosh of water. The floor of No 10 was damp.

I waited. A nurse came in with a tea-tray.

My bowels felt loose.

'How can I be sure of seeing Mr McMahon when he's finished operating?' I asked her.

'It's best to go over to the Theatre entrance. They usually confer afterwards. Then suddenly, they're gone. Over there, you'll be bound to catch him on his way out.'

'Thanks. I'll do that.'

. . . Jeff McMahon. Flecked amber eyes above the mask. Green-clad consultant surgeon. House surgeons. Theatre sisters. Shiny transparent gloves. Incisions. Clamps. Exploration. 'Look at this. See? It's spread to here. The lower intestine too. And the peritoneum's damaged drastically. He's a woeful mess!'

No! Think positively. It's a by-pass job. A satellite town built off the main motorway. By-pass and the traffic moves on . . .

I made a dash to the lavatory.

Half-an-hour passed. I carried the tray to the ward kitchen. The china tinkled in my trembling hands.

I sat on a window ledge opposite the Theatre doors. The corpse of a starling lay on the roof outside. A decomposing body on wet concrete; wings outstretched in cruciform; leaden with water.

Nathan had cautioned me. 'The most crucial time in surgery used to be during the operation. Anaesthetics were not what they are today. Now it's impossible to calculate where exactly the danger may lie. Robin's is such a complicated case that it's futile to contemplate it speculatively.'

Lunchtime. Mobile patients meandered towards the dining-room. The trim figure of Matron appeared. She joined me on the window seat.

'This is the hard time,' she said gently. 'The waiting.'

A pretty, neat woman of fifty plus, with soft silver hair. She had been at Bramble Grange since its foundation.

'You've seen so much. So many pass through here, Matron . . .'

She picked up my thoughts, looking towards the patients who drifted by. Several had facial disfigurements. Areas of skin marked in purple for treatment. Lumps and growths.

'Very many,' she agreed. 'What we give is time. And, to most people, time is valuable.'

At 1.00 p.m. a white-clad orderly ran up the stairs, two at a time. A Theatre nurse came out with oxygen cylinders. Together they went down in the lift and disappeared through a door marked 'Stores'. They reappeared with two more cylinders and vanished into the Theatre.

In the hall below, a little boy emerged. Perhaps three years old. A withered left arm; body dragging itself along the floor on his right buttock. The polished surface gave him added mobility. He reached up, kneeling. His face peered at the stairs above. He discovered a black aperture in a supporting column of the ceiling. Played 'Peep' with the footsteps that came and moved overhead and never reached his incumbent body. His laughter broke out in baby gurgles.

Cecil Kissane came from his Laboratory. Long easy strides.

'You're working a six-day week?' I commented.

'Duty calls,' he smiled readily. 'Actually, I'm here for Robin's results.' He moved on. 'I'll be with you in a minute.'

At the Theatre door, he met Dr Hunter; then continued into the operating precinct.

Dr Hunter came over. Theatre whites; green gown discarded. 'Wait here, Mrs Heron. Mr McMahon will be with you soon.'

I glanced at my watch. It was two and a half hours since I had arrived.

Cecil Kissane joined me. The same casual manner. 'I've just seen Robin. He's stood up extraordinarily well to surgery.'

Relief swamped me. 'Do you think there's much danger of further regeneration of activity in the gut? As a result of this operation, I mean, Cecil?'

His name slipped through from my subconscious.

'Personally, I don't,' he said candidly. 'Dr Monaghan is afraid of that, I know. No! I feel that even if it does happen, we may by then have an answer to this parasite. Robin's astonishingly healthy and surprisingly well.'

'I found a few silverfish in a food press in the kitchen. You know, those fast moving little sinuous things with tiny frail antennae? Lepismae, aren't they?'

'Don't worry. It's nothing like that. No! I think we're on to a nematode. We should know pretty soon.'

Jeff McMahon emerged. White mesh nylon vest, white trousers. His torso was hairy.

He took off gold-rimmed bi-focals and slipped them into his pocket. His face was relaxed. I noticed tiny broken veins on his cheeks.

He leaned beside me over the well of the stairs. Blue rails; chrome polished surface.

His words were cautiously confident. 'I'm quite pleased. The blockage was there. Smaller than I'd feared, but serious. I effected a by-pass.'

Warmth towards him emanated from me. It was almost physical. His arm, beside mine on the bannister rail, was brown-skinned and coated with tendrils of thick black hair. I felt an urge to touch it. I quashed the impulse. Western civilisation has conditioned us from spontaneous expression which could be subject to sexual interpretation. And part of his appeal for me, I acknowledged to be sexual.

'Did you find anything else, Mr McMahon?'

His face was only inches away from mine. The flecked eyes mesmeric. For the first time, I noticed his mouth. Slightly irregular teeth. I broke the embarrassment of blatant intimacy by looking away.

'Well, the condition of the peritoneum and intestines is very satisfactory. Much healthier than when I saw it internally, six weeks ago. I've put a small drain from the stomach instead of inserting a Ryle's tube. It will carry off the bile juice etcetera rather than Robin having the discomfort of that messy mucous in his mouth. Later it will be removed. This gastrostomy tube means, too, that nutriment can be fed that way – pushed up it.'

He had answered all my unvoiced questions.

He continued on a further note of hope. 'The smaller size of the blockage could mean that we're nearer the end of the parasitic infestation. Anyway, I've reinserted the drip in the same vein. I'm satisfied with that, for the moment.'

Robin came back on a Theatre trolley. Oxygen cylinders were strapped beneath it. An Aminsol drip was connected to his groin. A blood transfusion was ordered for later on.

He surfaced from the anaesthetic before I left. 'I want a bottle.' His voice was strong. A flood of urine came.

Sr Ryan was going off-duty. 'Isn't it great that the intestines are so good?' she said jubilantly.

Cecil Kissane was working in his Laboratory. The electric bulb cut a swathe of light on to the passage. His sandy head was bent over a table.

I went out into the rain.

*   *   *

Cecil Kissane was talking with Dr Hunter. He stopped me as I passed his Laboratory. Dr Hunter melted away.

Two days had passed since surgery.

'Robin's blood serum has gone to the Wellcome Laboratories. His antibodies are very active, healthy and resiliant. They will be tested against all parasites – and they've all the known ones over there.'

'In London?'

'Yes. There will be a response. And then we have the answer.' He sounded boyishly elated.

'So you're sleuthing the original cause, now? A parasite of some sort? And the bluebottle maggots – that business was secondary . . . ?'

'It was secondary but a fact,' he confirmed. He turned back to his Laboratory. 'Come in here a moment. I've something to show you.'

It was a small, clinically tidy room. Ovens, culture bowls, dishes. A folding table on which a microscope was mounted.

Cecil lifted down a glass phial. Inside, impaled on a pin like a tiny taxidermist's model, was an innocuous housefly.

Before he spoke, I knew its origin.

'The discharge from the fistula *did* contain a parasite. This chap is one of the cultures from it.'

Swab. Culture. Eggs. Grubs. Metamorphosis to – this!

'The bluebottle's legacy of activity is completely finished now. Mr McMahon is satisfied on that point and so am I. Only the parasite, the original cause of Robin's trouble, remains.'

Repugnance had vanished. Incredibly I felt a sympathy for the impaled insect. Laboratory specimen; induced; processed; living; speared to death by a pin; winged creature destined never to fly.

By showing it to me, Cecil Kissane had expunged the wraith of revulsion and quietly closed the chapter on a nightmare of horror.

Robin's spirits rose for a few days. He felt hungry and wanted roast beef and vegetables. He settled for three teaspoonfuls of tepid tea.

Then one afternoon, he started to whimper. Sr Ryan drew fluid off the stomach by unclipping the Meredith bag from the bed and placing it on the floor to drain. A few bubbles of flatulence dribbled out. Robin felt more comfortable.

Dr Monaghan checked his abdomen. 'Good. It's nice and soft.'

That night I noticed blood congealing in the gastrostomy tube.

Nurse Gilligan checked Robin's file. 'The day staff have registered rather large quantities of bile,' she said.

The blood flow increased. Robin lay breathing with slow panting exhalations.

Dr Hunter was called and he telephoned Jeff McMahon. He came back to No 10. 'Mr McMahon is satisfied that the blood is probably from internal sutures, or possibly an irritation where the tube enters the stomach. We're going to seal off the tube on the outside. This will give the new by-pass a trial chance to work.'

A cork stopper was plugged to the gastrostomy tube.

Next day, at regular intervals, the cork was removed and the fluid drained off. Scissors, with flat serrated edges like pliers, temporarily sealed it.

Bile juice came. It was clear of blood.

'Wellcome Laboratories are working hard,' Cecil Kissane said, 'and in the meantime, Robin's definitely better from my viewpoint. His haemoglobin is good and his antibodies are almost normal.'

'What's Wellcome's line of enquiry?' I asked.

'A nematode. I mentioned it to you as a possibility, a while back.' Behind the tinted glasses, his eyes were frank; unguarded.

'And that means . . . ?'

'Nematoda are a phylum of animals – that's a division – not closely related to any other. They include many free-living forms and plant parasites; like eelworm in potatoes. Or animal parasites – for example, the hook-worm. Actually, they've many peculiarities and variations in their excretory and reproductive systems, and in their muscular and body development.'

'And somewhere amongst them all may be something which has infested Robin's body?'

'That's what Wellcome Laboratories think is most likely.'

Five days after surgery, the drip slipped out from the vein. Robin's temperature rose – 102, 103. His bowels moved; a fluidic green matter. Four tablespoonfuls of water each hour, orally.

The portable X-ray unit was wheeled in again.

Just before midnight, Dr Hunter telephoned me at home. 'I had a night off and was out until now. We've a new problem as, being you, you'll probably have noted! We can feed a certain amount of nourishment intramuscularly. And we can push Complan up the gastrostomy tube. But that drip will have to go back into a vein. It's absolutely essential now for Robin. I'll do it tomorrow morning in Theatre. It's sterile over there. I just didn't want you to be alarmed if he's not in No 10 when you come in.'

Soft moaning. 'Leave me alone. Just leave me alone.'

The drip was attached in the area of the collarbone and held in place by strapping.

Robin's hands were shaking. His body trembling. On his right shoulder, a scimitar-shaped arc curved along the flesh from armpit to chest. The incision was held by ten stitches. A nurse covered it with a sterile dressing. It was garnet-edged in blood.

Temperature 104. Pulse slowing down. He looked dreadful.

The night-light bulb failed. An E.N.T. lamp stood temporarily in the corner, an extraordinary artefact like an old galleon's hurricane lamp.

The skin took on a yellow tinge. The jaundice began to return.

A couple of days later, Bob phoned Jeff McMahon.

'Robin is critical,' the surgeon said sombrely. 'The condition is disturbing and we haven't yet traced it.'

I left my mother with Robin one afternoon and took Billie and Helen up the hills with a couple of their friends. I packed a thermos for an impromptu picnic and tried to recreate the ruptured shell of family life. They played in a stream which opened into a clear shallow pool of mountain water. Carting stones and rocks, they built a dam.

A cool mist hung over the hills, but in the shelter of the valley, the sun was hot. An open quarry to the south hummed with mechanised activity. A red-haired Rolf Harris sat high up on his yellow cab, expertly scooping mounds of silver sand, and ferrying the load to a builder's truck which was waiting.

Tea-time. The quarry fell silent. The season's young lambs, independent now of maternal care, raced across the sloping field. A herd of Friesian calves wandered down to the pool, tails flicking off the hungry flies. Shafts of hazy sunlight filtered through a misty sky.

Peace suffused the valley.

... This is what Robin will be to me. Birdsong. River water. Soft hills. The things he once enjoyed. His memory will be, in time, a happy one. Good times that have gone. Robin: adventurous, observant, aware, sensitive.

And now I am here. And he is lying in a hospital bed, his grandmother keeping vigil by his side. Yet there is more of his spirit here than in the scarred body and terror-riddled mind. Perhaps, in his subconscious, in the twilight world of sleep, he's with us now. Empathy can transcend time and place ...

The tears came. Trickling at first, then spilling over. Flowing down my face, swelling my eyes to blotched red puffiness.

The children looked at me curiously: '*Grown-ups do not cry!*' They looked away.

Convulsively my whole frame began to shake.

I floated with the wave of tears until its tide drained dry.

EIGHT

September, October, November

'La verité est en marche; rien ne peut plus
l'arreter.'

Emile Zola (Article on the Dreyfus case)

'Look at them,' Robin held his hands outstretched. 'Just look. They're so weak and trembling. They'll never be right again.'

A blood count had been taken. A surgical pad covered the pierced skin. His eyes were twitching. He looked over his body objectively. The upper abdomen was becoming distended again; the blue veins reappearing.

I mentally totted-up the incisions. Seventeen drip insertions and surgical knifings.

Uncannily, he voiced my calculations. 'About seventeen, isn't it? Including the drips. Dead bark, that's all I am. I'll never be better.'

A nurse brought a concoction prescribed by Jeff McMahon. 'Can I gulp it down quickly?' Robin's voice was tetchy.

'No. Better take it in sips or it might make you vomit.'

The depression deepened. 'I'm desperately unhappy. I'll kill myself. I'm going mad and I can't do anything about it. I wish I was dead. I wish I'd never lived. I hate everything: toys, books, television – the lot. There's nothing but blackness; darkness. It's hopeless.'

I stood up uneasily and looked from the window. He was articulating my feelings with psychic accuracy.

The garden was ablaze with September colour. Vivid, bright, cruel colours.

His eyes glowered at me. 'If you leave this room, I'll tear up the sheets and smash up the place. I'll crawl out of bed and throw myself out of that window.' The voice grew stronger, homing in for the final sally. 'I've got my rights. I can kill myself if I want to. Voluntary Euthanasia you could call it . . .'

. . . Does one reach a sub-level of misery where nothing exists but this moment? This trapped world? This tortured body? Where all one's senses are dimmed to everything save conscious awareness of endless timeless suffering synthesised in this one moment . . . ?

I came back to the bed and took Robin's hand in silence.

Cecil Kissane proffered a theory.

'This situation, this acute depression, could be anaesthetic reaction. One sometimes gets it about a week after surgery. Admittedly, it's now over a fortnight since Robin's by-pass operation was done; but it's a possibility.'

'Is there any way to help him, Cecil?'

'It *is* a problem. He's had nothing but adult company for so long; and he's only a nine-year-old child, after all. As to the pain, well, they may be reducing the drugs. I just don't know.'

'How's your end of it going? The parasite?'

'We've all the stops out. Working on it.'

Robin started to vomit again.

Sr Ryan's optimism ebbed. 'It's such a diffused situation. And it's been too long for such a little chap; too much suffering. It's very sad, for he fights so hard. Sometimes, early in the morning, I notice him struggling to concentrate on reading; anything to distract himself and combat this depression business.'

Sips of Bovril.

'We're trying to get something into him orally. He seems to feel severe pain when we feed him through the gastrostomy tube,' Dr Hunter said.

The stitches were snipped out from the groin. Afterwards, Robin panicked. His eyes rolled; his breathing came in gasping punches. 'I . . . I . . . aye . . .' hissed out through clenched teeth.

God! What can I do? What can I do? 'Try to say it, Robin. What's wrong? We can help perhaps, if we know,' I pleaded.

'I'm beyond help. I'm going mad. I know I'm going mad.'

Like the old dog, I stumbled back to the stony road. But my zest was failing and my voice sounded weary and unconvincing.

'We have our minds, Robin. *You* know that. We'll always be free there. *You* told me that when things were worse than this, in Holy Innocents'.'

He whimpered his reply. 'No! Not any more. My mind is going too. There's only blackness. I'm going mad. Quite mad!'

A penumbra of conflicting facts. Where would it end?

*　　　*　　　*

An elderly man with a pleasant smile and rimless spectacles was a patient in No 12, the pink-papered room which had been Robin's the previous summer.

He frequently made sorties past No 10, en route to the toilet. Then he would reappear, walking slowly back to No 12. Although he never seemed to glance through Robin's open door, he must have noticed the colourful ornithology charts pinned to the walls because one morning a nurse arrived with a book on native wild birds.

'The patient in No 12 thought Robin might like to look at this,' she explained.

The fly-leaf bore the name 'Stephen O'Connor'. When Robin had finished perusing it, I laid it on his locker to return it when next I saw Mr O'Connor. But he didn't reappear.

One night, when the passage was quiet, I softly knocked on his door. It was opened by a tiny lady. Mr O'Connor was lying very still, propped up on pillows. An oxygen cylinder stood beside the bed. Another little lady sat in the corner; two little birds on a branch. Waiting; waiting. The Venetian blinds were closed.

Embarassed by my intrusion, I gave her the book and whispered my explanation and thanks.

A few minutes later, she pitter-pattered down the passage to Robin's room. She carried a paper-wrapped parcel in her hand.

'My husband asked me to buy this for your little boy,' she said. 'I brought it in today. But he's too poorly to give it to him, himself. We'd like your child to have it – from Stephen.'

It was an expensive battery-operated toy, chosen with thought and care. A long flex connected the controls to a feathered yellow bird. With the gentlest hand pressure, the bird hopped and sang a trill of music. It was the perfect selection for a child who loved wild creatures and whose fingers were too weak to constructively play with conventional toys.

I saw Stephen O'Connor's death notice in the newspaper a few days later.

The gold plumaged bird stood on Robin's trolley for many weeks. It reminded him of home; of pet animals; especially of Oblomova – his dachshund.

For me, it remained a tribute to the kindness of the suffering, for the suffering. It still sings. The golden bird.

En route to No 10, one morning a few days later, Cecil Kissane stopped me. His sensuous mouth was twisted in a glowing smile. 'I've something to tell you.'

We huddled in a corner like conspirators. Dr Hunter was telephoning from the Pathology Laboratory.

'Wellcome Laboratories have come up with a positive answer this morning. They've identified the parasite and told us of all the antigens.' His words tumbled on. 'I know Robin's not so good. Personally I feel that the rejaundicing of the liver could come from I.V. feeding rather than the chemical activity of the parasite. The damage from surgery wouldn't be permanent; no more than that which many people, and older people than Robin, have managed to overcome. Pathologically, he's good. If he can stay at this standard for another couple of weeks, we should be able to do the trick.'

What can one say when hope is handed back? The trembling started. I braced myself against the cold radiator.

Cecil went on. 'Look. We've a little skin test to do. I've to get the Laboratory ready for an analysis. We should be all set about mid-afternoon. Would you like me to tell Robin?'

I nodded. He hesitated; then spoke. 'I've a rather strange request for you. Robin has mentioned owning a dog.'

Nothing surprised me any more; but this almost did. 'Yes. We've a dachshund – Oblomova. She's about five years old.'

'Could you bring me a specimen of her faeces? There may be a link up here. This parasite is comparatively rare in Ireland. But not unheard of.'

'Oh, God, Cecil, I'm beginning to think we've a chance of winning through.' I was verging on tears. At Holy Innocents', it had been a lone battle against pain. At Bramble Grange, a combined struggle to sustain life. Now – at last – there was hope for a real future.

Cecil was beaming behind his tinted glasses. 'Dr Hunter will explain the clinical position to you. He's telephoning the Veterinary College now.'

I loitered outside the door while he went off to talk with Robin. Dr Hunter was still on the telephone when Cecil returned. He produced a pipe and laboriously started filling it from a worn pouch. There was an easy familiarity between us.

'You know, Bramble Grange is so different to the average hospital,' I ruminated. 'The fear structure doesn't exist here. The sort of situation where consultants are revered as oracles, I mean. Where the housemen are overworked and always in a hurry dealing with crises; and the nurses-in-training are in terror of the staff sisters. Here, it's a co-operative effort; and there's this extraordinary honesty, even about your divergence of views. It's very refreshing. I mean, although I sometimes may seem to be, I'm not completely asinine, and it's nice to be treated as if I've some I.Q.'

He puffed my self-deprecation aside in a cloud of smoke.

I went on. 'Here it isn't forgotten that each patient is an individual person. Not just a case or a number and name on a chart. Each is a unique part of humanity.'

He tapped the bowl of his pipe. 'It's rarely I get a chance to meet patients, you know. To me it would be too easy for them to become just names, specimens of tissue, urine and faeces.'

I looked at him squarely. 'You're a helluva team. Respect is something which has to be won. You've won ours.'

'Thanks. We try our best. But we make mistakes too.'

'And you're honest enough to admit it. That's a rare quality.'

Dr Hunter joined us. 'Cecil has filled you in?'

'As much as I'm capable of absorbing, yes.'

'Good! You're a great trouper.' The tangled skein of confusion was beginning to unwind. He went on. 'Look, I'm calling in an opthalmic specialist. It's to do with part of this parasitic infestation.'

I didn't ask him any details of that. Robin's eyes hadn't caused him any trouble. I latched on to the identity that had been established.

'Does it have a name? The infestation, I mean?'

'Of course. *Toxocara canis*. A dog parasite, actually.'

My audial memory was by now razor-edged. I noted the syllabic phonetic sounds for relay to Nathan.

Robin was reading when I came back that night. The skin test had not distressed him. He seemed to revive and respond to activity.

'Another doctor came this evening. They called him "Doctor"

though he was a surgeon. Dr Hunter explained that opthalmic surgeons are called "Doctor" to distinguish them from general surgeons. Medicine's a complicated thing, isn't it?'

'What did he do?'

'Dr Ferris, you mean?' He was nonchalant. 'Well, he had a little torch and he looked into both my eyes. I don't know what they'll be up to next. But anyway, he was a very nice chap. He'll come again, he said.'

I was puzzled. Robin hadn't complained of impaired vision. However, Dr Hunter spoke to me before he went off-duty. 'Dr Ferris is a consultant surgeon in the Royal Elizabeth Eye and Ear Hospital. He was a G.P. actually, before he specialised; and he's a very competent man. He may bring some equipment here to Bramble Grange to give him a better idea of what's happening. But there's definitely some Toxocara activity behind the left eye. However, we're fairly confident that the condition throughout the whole body can be treated with drugs. Treated completely and effectively.'

Next day, Robin was lifted from bed and seated in a chair for a couple of hours. His abdomen and trunk were distended and tight as a tambourine. The drip was playing up again. It was reinserted in his left hand and reinforced by a splint.

Professor O'Grady came down to the sitting-room. 'The best I can say is that it's more hopeful.'

'He's still having considerable pain.' My words reverberated like a muezzin's familiar cry.

'I agree with you there. And I also believe it's genuine.'

'He seems to be hitting terrible troughs of depression, Professor.' I sounded like a meterologist forecasting a wet weekend.

I baited another line and cast it. 'Do you think he'll make a complete recovery to health, or will he be delicate for life – assuming he pulls out of this?'

'We'll see about that when he's better,' he said, rather abruptly. Then, as though regretting the acidity of his reply, he softened his tone. 'Children don't have much resistance but they have remarkable resilience, you know.'

The weekend brought complications with the protesting drip. The fluid seeped into the tissue, swelling over the strapping on Robin's hand. The drip was removed and the oral intake doubled.

The pain grew more intense.

I vacillated between hope for a long-term future and the actuality of living out each minute of agony.

Oblomova took her regular journey from her basket to the shrubbery. I watched. Presently, she heaved her long body upwards and arched it against a trailing branch. Armed with a shovel, I scooped the steaming faeces into a polythene bag, sealing it with plastic wire. I then inserted it into another layer of polythene and wrapped it all in brown paper.

I was sweating and gagging by the time I had wiped the shovel clean. I attached a label: '*Dachsund excrement. Dog: property of Robin Heron. No 10. Ward P. Bramble Grange*'.

Cecil took it with a sardonic smile.

The pain situation was growing intolerable. Bob had a week's holiday and took over the morning visiting session.

After a lunch of jelly, the familiar bouts started. Robin was given an injection. It didn't work. Bob rang the bell.

'I don't think we can do anything else,' a nurse said apologetically.

Another ten minutes elapsed. Robin was writhing; shrieking.

Bob went to the Station. 'Isn't there anything to alleviate this pain business?' he asked. 'Just a "Yes" or "No" – please!'

Sr Ryan was off-duty. The senior ward nurse answered uneasily. 'It's "No", I'm afraid.'

'Well then, could I speak to Dr Hunter?'

'Right,' she replied with relief. 'I'll have him bleeped.'

The chubby figure appeared within minutes. Bob was quietly assertive in his own courteous but positive way.

'The problem is the drugs, Dr Hunter,' he began. 'Now I'm aware that Robin must be a considerable nuisance . . .'

'Not at all,' Dr Hunter dissented politely.

Bob smiled. 'Don't give me that line.' They mutually dropped the pretence. Bob continued. 'If you had a little old lady sitting up there getting radium each morning, it would be much easier on all the staff.'

Dr Hunter shrugged. Then the spontaneous grin broke through.

'You're right, of course. Now look, Mr Heron, you could put it like this. We're being cruel to be kind. To be honest, it *is* possible to kill the pain completely with drugs by practically knocking Robin out into sleep. But the disadvantages are two-fold.'

Bob waited.

'First, the toxic effect of these drugs. Secondly, the enlarged condition of Robin's liver. It's now the size of an adult's, and this enlargement is undoubtedly causing pressure and consequently continuous pain. One of the ways to reduce the liver size is movement. Sitting, walking – as much normal physical activity as possible. If Robin is heavily drugged, this movement will be impossible and the liver will be considerably less likely to reduce in size. You're with me?'

'Yes. And – thanks! It's easier to take when one understands it.'

Dr Hunter turned to a positive theme. 'Actually, I'm going to get Robin up and moving tomorrow. Then we'll see about resuming physiotherapy.'

Robin awkwardly manoeuvred himself up. He was eased into his socks and sandals, stained with sea-spray. He was put sitting on the edge of his bed to swing his legs from the knees. Sweat stood out in beads on his face.

Two nurses linked him, their elbows locked under his arms. He let his weight rest on his feet. Took a wavering step. Then another. A third. His feet looked big and splayed as a limbo dancer's. He reached the chair and sat down, shaking with exhaustion. His face was flushed with colour.

'Now, when he's rested, Mrs Heron, we want you to encourage him to exercise his hands and feet as best he can.'

On their instructions, I slipped off the sandals and socks.

A tiny frail saffron-skinned wraith, he sat – fingers and toes clawing the empty air in an ersatz dog paddle.

Within days, the final inheritance of surgery was removed. The abdominal stitches were snipped and lifted out with tweezers. The drip changed hands again. His food intake increased but he vomited occasionally.

Cecil Kissane came down to No 10. He had heard news from the

Veterinary College. 'I sent the faeces out. I've enough of the human variety to deal with,' he added wryly, 'but the results from your dog were negative. She's clear of infection. *Toxocara canis* was not present. We were anxious to establish that as a precaution since you have other children.'

'How might Robin have picked up the parasite?' I asked.

He scratched a knobbly finger between the buttons of his psychedelic shirt. 'From what I'm learning of it, the infestation is in the puppy, often pre-natally there. It's less common in adult dogs. Mature toxocaral worms measure three to five inches. The eggs are discharged, sometimes in faeces. I suppose Robin could have got it anywhere – possibly sucking a blade of grass, or unconsciously ingesting them on contaminated fingers. Maybe handling a football that had rolled in dog excrement. Or uncooked vegetables, like lettuce. Pretty well anywhere.'

'And then?'

'Well, the pattern in man is that once ingested, the larvae develop from the eggs in the human intestine. A week after infestation in man, they are only 0.02 cm in diameter. They then develop to their second stage, with mouth parts and alae, or a type of wings. They penetrate the walls of the bowel and are carried in the blood to other parts of the body. The size to which a larva grows seems to determine its course of migration. They leave the blood vessels when they find the diameter of the channel constrictive on their bodies. Then they settle and form granuloma in the affected tissues.'

'And these tiny tumours were assumed to be malignant growths?'

'That's it,' Cecil agreed. 'But you do have to remember that it's a condition more common in warmer climates. Only seven cases of infestation had been identified in Britain in 1960 when the *British Medical Journal of Opthalmology* published a paper on it.'

Again the reference to opthalmic infestation. I decided to let it pass and discuss it with Nathan.

Cecil was still speaking. 'You know, to date, there are only two verified cases in Ireland. And there's another thing; one advantage to the victim is – though it makes diagnosis more difficult – the larvae never develop beyond this stage in man. They cannot reproduce themselves, as they do in dogs.'

'So, hopefully, once you've flushed them out, then that should be the end of them?'

'It's more than a hope. It's a fact.'

Hope seemed to surround No 10. Sr Ryan confided, 'You know, I think Robin will make it. It's as though he senses it himself. We have him sleeping at night now with just one tablet.'

But, inevitably, hope jack-knifed. Another fistula formed.

Jeff McMahon examined him and joined me in the sitting-room. 'Unfortunately, when I thought we were round the corner a few days ago, the vomiting started again. We're not out of the wood yet. That fistula has burst out the waste from the intestines. Surgery is impractical at the moment. The front abdominal wall is very inflamed. It's not a classical surgical situation where you remove the affected intestine and suture healthy pieces together. The problem of the Toxocara sees to that!'

The tawny eyes looked out to the garden. The square-tipped fingers drummed the window ledge. I was conscious again of his sexuality; of the dark hairs on his hands.

'This parasite is not complicated in treatment, you know. Just a matter of drugs; in humans, a response to these tablets we're giving him now. We're certain, too, of activity in the left eye. It usually shows up first in the eyes. Sometimes as a suspected retinablastoma.'

'And that is – what, Mr McMahon?'

He explained it was a tumour of the retina – the membrane which lines the back of the eye and is light-sensitive. He went on. 'These Toxocara tumours give considerable difficulty in identification, although, of course, they can be revealed by specialised tests.'

'Like the skin test which Robin has had?'

'That – and other techniques.'

'There's nothing for me to do or say, Mr McMahon. "They also serve who only stand and wait." That seems to have been our role for so long. So very long.'

Nathan started to ferret out what information he could.

'You know, Inez, you can't afford to be unrealistic – even though things augur well. The Toxocara could continue its travels to the brain. If so, the end could be very quick and unexpected.'

'But Robin's sitting out in a chair each day. Starting to walk . . .'

'Good, good,' he interjected. 'I only say that to warn you. I haven't seen Robin. I can only judge by what you tell me. However, I'll do some researching for you.'

That night I wrote to the Department of Zoology at a prestigious English university, and told them of Robin's history. I quoted from the *British Medical Dictionary* (1961) which referred to *Toxocara canis* infestation as having occurred 'rarely in man'. A reply came promptly. It was very courteous, sympathetic – and succinct. It stated that there was possibly some degree of inaccuracy in suggesting that this roundworm disease occurred 'rarely in man'. It was probably much more common than realised but might often be incorrectly diagnosed. The letter made reference to various Papers published on the subject and helpfully informed me how I could set about tracing them.

I passed the letter on to Nathan.

One evening he presented me with the photostat copy of one of the British medical journals. It had been published in September 1970 – twelve months earlier. An article in the journal dealt with Toxocaral infection; the disease, Toxocariasis, caused by *Toxocara canis*. There were some photographic illustrations.

He untangled the technical language and explained it to me. The last lines of the articles blazoned themselves in my mind . . . that Toxocariasis was scarcely known as a human infection until 1960 . . . that it is widespread and sometimes a cause of death . . . that the public health problems of the infection are grave and need prompt attention.

Again Robin began to slip back . . .

'I think he's failing,' Nurse Gilligan said sadly.

Sr Ryan confirmed it. 'Medically, he's pretty bad, I'm afraid.'

Dr Hunter was on the passage one evening. 'I've been lying in wait for you,' he said.

My body was weighted with weariness. He pulled up a chair for me in the sitting room.

'I've two things to tell you. First, Robin's antibodies are still virile and good. But secondly,' he paused for a moment, 'his liver is enlarged

– and that's very bad. He is extremely wasted. If we stopped nutriment through the I.V. feeding and took him off the drip, it's unlikely he'd last a week. He's vomiting up everything he takes orally. We've tried Vamin and stronger nutriment through the drip, but unsuccessfully.'

'The veins are giving trouble again, aren't they?' I had passed through the crucible. Mental exhaustion was draining me of hope; even of despair.

'They're very poor,' he admitted. 'We tried twice this afternoon to shift that drip. We tried the leg and the arm but we couldn't find a responsive vein. They're tired. As to the vomiting? It *may* be caused by feeding through the gastrostomy tube; or, more possibly, by the condition of the liver.'

'Dr Hunter, the left eye has a film across it.' With him, I didn't have to feign optimism. The weariness tinctured my voice.

'Yes. I noticed blood in it today. But it's not appreciably worse though it's becoming visible now. The treatment of the Toxocariasis has appeared to make some improvement. But it hasn't done all we had hoped for. As against that, we haven't been able to complete the treatment because of Robin's low state.'

Fatigue drowned me. I sat silent. Inert.

He stood up and gently helped me to my feet.

I walked back to No 10.

Day by day, Robin sank lower and lower. Slowly his head would turn, watching expressionless from the pillow. Seeing Bob. Seeing me. Seeing and unseeing.

Often during the daytime, I thought he was sleeping – so still he lay. But he was awake. Eyes now closed; now open, staring into nothingness.

The drip was inserted in his neck. Nutriment from two sources: Sterivac through the gastrostomy tube, Vamin fed into the vein.

Sunken eyes. Great black shadows beneath the protruding yellowed eyeballs. Fully conscious, but subhuman. Only his trembling hands, continuously shaking, showed signs of life.

I travelled beyond tears.

Beyond emotion.

Beyond caring.

I felt like baling out.

Like a sinking ship longing to desert the mice.

I sat, incarcerated in my own exhaustion. Hour after hour.

Day by day.

Bob voiced it one evening as I shuffled beside him to the car park. 'At the end of all that crisis of surgery, we seem to be back where we started.'

Zombie-like, I dropped into the passenger seat. 'I'm almost too jaded to care any more. I've nothing left physically or emotionally on which to draw. It would be easier for Robin, for all of us, if he was dead. If he had died months and months ago.'

Bob took my hand. 'I know. I know.'

Psychiatric suicide.

Emptiness.

Nothing but emptiness. "Too long a sacrifice can make a stone of the heart."

Inexplicably, Robin rallied again. With his extraordinary resilience, he lurched back from the brink and started to eat. Yoghurt, cheese and crackers. There was only occasional vomiting. No one attempted to explain it. They settled for capitalising on the capricious turn of fate. My energy began to filter back too. Apathy died.

Dr Monaghan encouraged Robin to sit out in a chair for a while each day.

One afternoon, as Jeff McMahon's car pulled in under the trees, Robin leaned near to the window and waved down to him, shouting 'Hi!'

The surgeon gave me a fillip. 'His liver is almost back to normal and his bowels are moving. I intend to give him a drug. It has proved satisfactory with this parasitic larvae in man. And it's in use in the U.S.A. and Britain.'

'Will it be prolonged treatment? I mean, Robin seems to swing from highs to lows?'

'One single day's dose is enough.'

Robin's basic maintenance was paid weekly. As yet, we had no idea of what drugs, tests, surgery, pathology, drips, etcetera might cost. We were partially covered by our contribution to the Voluntary Health Insurance Scheme. But obviously reimbursement would come nowhere near meeting the full expenses incurred.

It was the least concern on our minds at the moment. But Dr Hunter, in his pragmatic way, broached the subject. 'I understand you've a family connection with the pharmaceutical trade?'

'Yes. My brother-in-law.'

'Good,' he beamed. 'Now I've been talking to Cecil. He's putting through most of the laboratory tests on Robin as Research. That should help. As to maintenance, I think you should have a word with our Almoner. She'll guide you how to make application through the correct channels for special assistance. In cases of prolonged and extremely expensive illness – as Robin's is proving to be – the Department of Health sometimes views the situation very sympathetically; particularly with children. And, you know, if Robin pulls through – and we're more optimistic now – it would be a long time before he's completely off medication. It's no harm to open negotiations. As to the drips – some of them are very costly. You could make arrangements, if you like, to supply your own bottles. I'll give you an idea of what I'll need.'

I muzzled tears of appreciation.

He continued. 'You'll find, I think, that Professor O'Grady and Mr McMahon will settle for whatever your coverage is under the V.H.I. Scheme.' The boyish smile broke through. 'Sorry to be so mundane. It was just a thought, in case the extraordinarily heavy expenses were worrying you.'

'Thank you, Dr Hunter. It's kindness that touches me most of all. The pain, the suffering – they send the adrenalin coursing. But it's kindness like yours, when you view Robin not just as a case, but with a compassion that embraces us all – that's what moves me.'

My voice shook. But it had to be said.

We owed it to him. To them all.

Nurse Gilligan was tidying up Robin for the night, smoothing the sheets, applying a silver paste to his abdominal wound. Night Sister came in. I left for the sitting-room. She preferred it that way.

Suddenly there was an emergency. Nurse Gilligan's voice had a note of urgency. 'Robin! Robin! Can you hear me?'

Night Sister walked quickly down the passage.

The house phone dialled. 'Dr Hunter?'

Within minutes he came from the residency block.

The chaplain appeared.

An oxygen cylinder was trundled into No 10.

From the open door I heard words '... the pupils? Are they dilating?'

'He's in a coma ...'

'No response ...'

Someone closed the door.

Twenty sweating minutes passed. By degrees, they emerged. Dr Hunter came last. He spoke quietly. 'Robin was unconscious. We can't trace the exact cause. Tomorrow, we'll do a cardiograph.' His voice was subdued.

Next morning, I noticed a portable apparatus in the corner. A cardiograph machine. It looked innocuously like a record player. We didn't hear any results of the readings. But, by degrees, different theories were suggested as to the possible cause of the coma. Dr Monaghan felt it might be a tiny dead Toxocara mite in the bloodstream which had travelled to the brain and moved on. Cecil Kissane thought the interaction of so many drugs could have been a factor.

I dismissed it from my mind as Robin recovered from that unexplicable setback. He was taken off the drip. Before lunch, he drank a brandy and soaked it up with potatoes and minced beef. Gradually his colour improved. He started to read. His bowels moved.

Professor O'Grady gave his judgment. 'The jaundice is certainly much better. Almost gone.'

Warm mellow October days. A summer reluctant to pass, and Robin's sitting-up periods lengthened. 'It's time we got you out of doors again, Robin,' Dr Monaghan said.

The wheelchair routine of the previous year began once more.

... Copper leaves. Auburn rustling on a panned-out blue sky. Even the jackdaws sounded lazy. The magpies desultory in their chatter; pent-up energies spent. Soft drone of indolent insects; faint whisper of faraway traffic . . .

Several days passed without pain, without vomiting. Robin's left eye grew angrier in appearance.

A blood test was taken. Dr Hunter commented, 'The veins are showing up well. It's a lot easier to take blood.'

Robin was triumphant. 'I've had a few days with no injections at all. Things are definitely getting better, aren't they?'

Jeff McMahon endorsed it. 'I'm very pleased,' he said with under-statement.

One morning, two nurses arrived with a camera and tripod. Robin wriggled out of his pyjamas, as requested, and obligingly posed naked. They were chatty girls, interested in their assignment.

'These photographs are wanted for record purposes. To note Robin's progress.'

Though many battles had been lost, the war was being won.

Physiotherapy recommenced. Robin's legs and feet gradually strengthened. Shuffling steps grew in confidence. Soon he could walk alone, a lurching figure balancing with his arms and spindly legs.

He was weighed. The needle swung unsteadily; then settled, registering 40 lbs. It was the 'average' weight of a four-year-old child. He was now only days short of his tenth birthday.

His face was cadaverously thin. Jeff McMahon interpreted it with-out concern. 'The steroids puff out the features. Now that we've reduced them, naturally he looks much worse.'

'And the *Toxocara canis*?'

'Robin's had a major dose of the drug. The parasite has completely cleared from everywhere except the eye. And the hardness in his abdomen is gradually reducing,' he added encouragingly.

Robin sipped a medicinal sherry as an aperitif to his lunch. Sr Ryan poured some liquid from a bottle.

'This will stimulate the digestive functions and increase your appetite,' she said, as Robin looked charily at the spoon. 'Now we don't want to have to put you back on the drip when you're doing so well. But you're going to have to try and eat and drink everything we give you. It really is important, Robin,' her musical voice coaxed.

*   *   *

His tenth birthday passed at Bramble Grange. Again friends rallied round with cards and presents. Again the cook sent up a cake alight with candles.

Dr Monaghan sounded a fresh note of optimism. 'Hi, soldier! Happy birthday! Soon we're going to think of getting you home in the afternoons.'

Next day, Robin's eye was angry and bloodshot. Within hours, it had deteriorated and narrowed to a slit.

Dr Ferris called. I didn't meet him. But that night, Dr Hunter reported the findings. 'There's an increase of activity in the left eye. In time, this will regress but it has damaged the vision – to what degree Dr Ferris can't accurately estimate without full apparatus, lights, etcetera.'

'So he may be blind in that eye ultimately?' I wanted a denial.

'It's possible, yes.' He didn't lie.

'Robin doesn't seem to have noticed that his sight is impaired. He's conscious only of the pain.'

'That's because the other eye has adjusted to the situation. Remember it's happened gradually. But the damaged eye *is* encysted.'

Two facial X-rays were taken.

It was decided to treat the affected eye with radium. Robin was wheeled down to the Therapy Department. The staff greeted him enthusiastically. Dr Monaghan marked the skin with purple triangles.

The treatment was brief and caused no nausea or pain. But afterwards, Robin rebelled. 'I hate hospitals and everything in them. I don't want any more doctors looking at me; poking at me. I want nothing but just to ease the pain of this bloody eye,' he said grouchily.

It was balm to hear him fighting back.

He had moved forward from apathy; away from passive acceptance of the inevitable. He was taking a truculent stand. When he was angry, he expressed it verbally – sometimes without diplomacy. But everyone was tolerantly indulgent.

Cecil Kissane came to the rescue. As Robin see-sawed along the passage one day, Cecil called him into the laboratory.

Robin was fascinated. 'I saw some of those little dishes in which he cultures bacteria. Then he puts the dishes into a glass-fronted oven and presses a control switch. Cecil let me do it, too. He put a plate under a microscope and let me see a hair; and he showed me tissues and blood cells.'

I carried Robin from the car into the house. It was Billie's birthday, and Robin had come home to celebrate with the family. He looked even worse than in hospital. An eye-shield covered the blood-bathed cornea. His clothes dangled shapelessly from his emaciated body. But he was elated.

Home became a daily outing.

One night, after Robin had been settled back to bed in Bramble Grange, Dr Ferris called. I was heading through the door of No 10, carrying a urinal bottle to the sluice room. We almost collided.

'Put that weapon down and stay a moment,' he smiled. 'I'll need you to give Robin moral support.'

He was a big muscular man. Dark-skinned, with the physique of a boxer in training. His touch had the gentleness of the very strong for the very weak.

Softly his fingers rested on Robin's eyes. 'Now, Robin. See if you can open this one.' His index finger lingered on the left lid. 'Try it yourself; or, if you like, I'll help you.'

Whimpering with pain, Robin eased open the damaged eye. It was a bloodshot mess.

'You're a great lad. Okay! Relax now. I'm not going to do anything more to you. We're going to clear that up. Not to worry. Right?'

Robin gave a watery grin.

Dr Ferris walked up the passage with me, attuning his wide stride to mine. He stopped at the Station, safely out of Robin's listening range. 'You're his mother?'

'Yes.' My voice sounded a trembling falsetto.

'You've had two dreadful years. Dr Hunter has filled me in on all that's happened.'

I nodded. 'We have. And we've got used to hearing the truth, Dr Ferris. Even when it's very bad. We appreciate the honesty of those who are frank with us, as everyone has been here at Bramble Grange. So please tell me what you think.'

'I will. That eye is very very sore. Radiation probably has not aggravated it – it possibly would have regressed anyway. But the primary aim is to alleviate pain. The Toxocara is dead. Quite dead now in the eye. And, as you know, it's completely gone from all other parts of the body. That chapter of activity is over.' He continued. 'I'm going to prescribe treatment. But if the pain persists, I'll have to do a diathermy on it.'

Nathan pulled a chair close to the fire.

'It's question time as usual, Nathan. What's a diathermy?'

'It means passing an electric needle in to the root of the trouble. It's the production of heat in tissue to relieve symptoms of inflammation or pain. A high-frequency current.'

'It sounds awful. Do you imagine it could be done at Bramble Grange?'

'I think it's unlikely, Inez. It could need quite complex equipment, I think. But it may not come to that, remember. After all, Dr Ferris has prescribed treatment. That may work.'

He looked very old and very tired. I felt a guilt for all the draining I had done on him for so long. A wave of affection flooded out of me.

'Nathan, I don't know how I'd have got through all this without you. I've leaned so much on your loyalty to me, on your knowledge and strength in these awful months. You do know that I'm more grateful than I can ever say?'

'I know. I know, Inez. But you've made me feel useful. That's important. To feel needed; wanted. Even to have someone call me by my Christian name. As one grows older there are fewer and fewer people around to do that.' He gestured to an unfinished canvas. 'I'm going away for a couple of weeks. Going south. A bit of sketching I want to do before the winter really sets in. I'll be in touch with you as soon as I get back.'

A postcard came from Kerry a few days later.

Nathan never returned.

He died suddenly. A heart attack.

There was no one to whom I could write the conventional letter of sympathy.

I wrote words. Final words. To Nathan. To myself . . .

'. . . I am glad I spoke those last thoughts to you when I did. Broke the reticence that binds feelings which are real. When I heard of your passing, I cried. Not just tears – but a drenching from my heart. And still I am blinded by unshed tears when I think of you. Pass your home. I wanted to call; if anyone was there, to ask for one of your paintings, a book, anything. But no! I do not need mementos to remember you. For me, you will always live in memory.

Perhaps that is the most any of us can expect of immortality. That we live on in remembrance in the minds of those who have loved us.

So it shall be for me. Dear Nathan. Beloved friend.

Goodbye . . .'

Hallowe'en passed. The shops gay with masks, balloons and bright cartons of nuts.

On school's half-term holiday, Billie and Helen shyly came to Bramble Grange to visit Robin. He hadn't been home for a few afternoons.

November days. The eye drops were an anathema to Robin. He winced and pulled away as they were inserted. 'I'm going to kick that bloody doctor in the face. I hate these things.'

Gently, Sr Ryan prised open the inflamed lid. The dropper ejected its prescribed allocation of fluid. Shuddering tears. Knobbly knees drawn up to quivering chin in reflex reaction to pain. He hugged his legs to stop himself from the prohibited motion of wiping away the excess liquid from his eyes.

I sat by the bed. He reached out and felt blindly for my hand. Then he raised his head. 'My poor old eye.'

My composure broke. I cried. Tears for Robin. For Nathan. For Bob and myself. For the backlash of over a year of exhaustion and drained emotion.

'Robin, what are we going to do?'

'There's nothing we can do, Mum. And, anyway, this old eye is clearing up. Look! the bottle says "3 drops daily" – and it's nearly npty now. I'll soon be home again for keeps. You'll see.'

Roles of comforter reversed.

The treatment worked. The pain diminished and died.

Robin came home again for the afternoons' outings and had tea
ith us before returning to Bramble Grange. He was looking better
d growing stronger.

Great heavy-headed chrysanthemums. An end-of-summer fragrance
me. Nurse Gilligan carried a vase from a patient's room. 'I loathe the
tumn,' she said. 'No wonder they call it the Fall in the States. It's the
d of everything.'

'I know. But somehow, this year – for us – I think it's just the
ginning. A new beginning.'

Dr Monaghan was thinking on the same lines. 'We're going to try
ting Robin home overnight. We'll give you tablets for the treat-
ent of pain, should you run into trouble on that score.'

Sr Ryan made the arrangements. 'We'll hold Robin's room for a
w days, just in case he needs it.'

A porter wheeled him out to the car.

It was five months since we had made the nightmare journey from
sclahane.

But the overnight trial was successful. Robin slept. A deep peaceful
ep. No moaning. No restlessness. Next day, he had a bath.

The long slow haul back to living had begun.

few days later, I returned to pack Robin's suitcase.

It was Sunday morning. The car park was deserted. The blinds
sed on the window of the Pathology Laboratory.

I sat for a while looking out on the garden. The asters had been
ared from the soil. Neat rows of wallflowers awaited spring's
vival.

During the night a tree had fallen. Its tortured branches ploughed
o the earth. Grotesque roots reached skeletal fingers to the
es.

A quixotic breeze swept the dying leaves up in a whirlpool of
otion. A macabre ballet of amber, russet, gold. Some shivered and
ng on. Some broke free and drifted away. Some fluttered to the
ound – and lay still.

In life, there are the victims. And the survivors.

I closed the suitcase.

On the wall was a giant poster of Pinnochio, the puppet boy who came to life.

I left it there.

EPILOGUE

'. . . that most inspiring of human
qualities – the capacity to endure and
to keep one's form against overwhelming
odds.'
Harold Hobson

even years have passed.

Robin is sixteen now.

He lost the vision in the infected eye and is now blind in the left ye forever.

His scarred body has healed. He is limited, to an extent, by the eritage of his damaged health and he lacks stamina. He retained his nterest in ornithology and fishing – and has become an enthusiastic hotographer. He reads extensively and has recently started playing olf and cycling. At the moment, he is studying for his Honours eaving Certificate at school, and plans to go to university to take a egree in Micro-biology.

His time in the limbo-land of suffering lost him his childhood; but e gained a maturity far beyond his chronological age – a maturity vhich many adults never achieve.

The trauma of the past is now a fading memory to him, and his uture stretches to wide and far horizons.

s for me?

Those shadowed years were my metamorphosis. My initial resent-nents have subtly changed. I now feel only a terrible sadness that so nuch suffering could, perhaps, have been avoided.

My childhood's legacy of unquestioning acceptance of authority and onvention is jettisoned. I've established my own code of integrity by hich I live. And I have found myself as an individual.

Today, I sincerely believe in legalised Voluntary Euthanasia.

Although I lost my faith in God and man's immortality, I have arned to survive without dependence on supernatural help or omfort.

Physicians and surgeons I now see as scientists and technicians – ighly trained men. But, with the aura of medical mystique removed, ey seem to me to vary – as all people do – in their abilities, their edication, and their compassion.

Robin was lucky – and we were lucky too – that, at Bramble Grange, we found a team who would not accept defeat. We owe them a debt which can never be repaid for they gave the gift of life. They won because they refused to lose.

FOR THE LOVE OF ANN
James Copeland

'The doctor cleared his throat and spoke very quietly. "I am so sorry to have to tell you this, but I'm afraid that our tests show that it is extremely unlikely that your daughter will ever be educated, or for that matter, that she will ever be able to recognize you as her parents." '

That was in 1958 and Ann Hodges was six years and eight months old. Today that same girl is in her twenties, full of charm, devoted to her parents and her brothers and excitedly taking in the world and its challenges.

Between those two dates lies a remarkable story. A love story born out of hopelessness and ignorance and nurtured in years of tears and joy . . .

ALL FOR THE LOVE OF ANN

55p

A BREATH OF BORDER AIR
Lavinia Derwent

'Looking back, I often wonder if any of it was real . . .'

Lavinia Derwent, well known as a best-selling author of children's books, and as a television personality, memorably portrays a childhood spent on a lonely farm in the Scottish Border country.

Hers was an enchanted world of adventure: a world of wayward but endearing farm animals, and of local characters like Jock-the-Herd . . . and Lavinia's closest friend, Jessie, who never failed to temper her earthy wisdom with a rare sense of humour.

'A love of a book' *Glasgow Herald*

60p

HOW TO ORDER

If you would like to order any of the books advertised in these pages, send purchase price plus 8p postage per book to Arrow Books, Book Service by Post, P.O. Box 29, Douglas, Isle of Man. Customers outside the UK should send purchase price plus 10p postage per book.

Whilst every effort is made to keep prices down and to keep popular books in print, Arrow Books cannot guarantee that prices will be the same as those advertised here or that the books will be available.